SORRY FOR THE WEIGHT

ARIEL D. BAKER CPT, MSN RN

As Told To
NICOLE D. MILLER

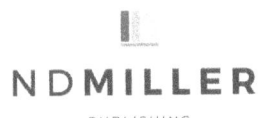

Copyright © 2025 by Ariel D. Baker, CPT, MSN RN

All rights reserved by the author. No part of this book may be reproduced or used in any manner without written permission of the copyright owner (author) except for the use of quotations in a book review. The author guarantees all contents are original and do not infringe upon the legal rights of any other person or work. For more information, address: info@ndmillerpublishing.com.

ISBN: 978-1-7352735-6-3

Editing by Piper Youtzy

Book cover design by Sherita Carthon

Ghostwritten by Nicole D. Miller

Disclaimer: The names of many individuals in this book have been changed. The descriptions and reflections are meant to be impressions and opinions of the Author's experiences. This book contains depictions of eating disorders, intimate partner violence, and other themes that some readers may find disturbing.

To my son, the miracle baby.

Contents

Chapter 1 *Apple Jacks*	1
Chapter 2 *Field Day*	8
Chapter 3 *Mean Girls*	14
Chapter 4 *Fly Girl*	22
Chapter 5 *Track Star*	31
Chapter 6 *Baby Mama*	41
Chapter 7 *Miracle Baby*	52
Chapter 8 *Porcelain White*	62
Chapter 9 *Red Flag*	70
Chapter 10 *Big Stepper*	81
Chapter 11 *The Rebrand*	92
Acknowledgments	103

Chapter 1
APPLE JACKS

"And the Line Leader of the week is——Ariel!" my first-grade teacher, Ms. S., announced proudly to the class.

Wow! Me?!

Excitement flushed my chipmunk cheeks as a large smile stretched them beyond measure. In no time, I had leapt to my feet from my desk in my light pink velour shorts and white tee, ready to lead the class to the gymnasium.

Being the Line Leader for the week was a big deal. It meant I had completed all my assignments last week, gotten to school on time, and had all-around good behavior. It was a badge of honor that I eagerly wore.

Chairs scratched the linoleum floor and were shoved against the desks as students scurried from a blob into a line so Ms. S. could count us before we headed out. My chin held a slight lift to it, knowing that *I* was the one who would be *first* once we got into place. But soon after, butterflies began flapping in my stomach. On my way to my destination at the front, I had to pass *him*. My very first crush. TJ. TJ was one of the most popular boys in class. Hershey's chocolate skin, hair-faded with a long rat-tail dangling in the back, and always Nautica and Fubu'd down from head to toe. That boy was fine! And the best part was he smelled just like my favorite cereal: Apple Jacks.

TJ saw me comin' and did something that made me melt. He smacked the back of my bare legs, causing skin-to-skin contact.

He touched me! I nearly fainted.

My already amazing day had gone from great to even better. That morning, I had specifically chosen my outfit thinking of TJ and knew I was cute. The fact that he flirted in his 7-year-old way confirmed it. I floated to the front of the line on cloud nine while planning our future wedding. But then, whispers and snickers from behind stopped me dead in my tracks.

What's going on? I wondered, a sense of dread slowly emerging as I strained my ears to listen.

"You know she likes you," one of the popular girls sneered at TJ.

My heart beat a little faster. My secret crush wasn't as much of a secret as I thought. I turned around and saw that the culprit who outed me was the "light-skin-long-hair-don't-care" type. You know, the ones that all the boys liked. The fly girls with their Clorox-white bobby socks bouncing in rhythm to their mixed curls. I could tell by her tone the girl's intent was malicious, but it wasn't even her statement that would do the most damage to my young self-esteem. It was TJ's response.

"I can't like her! She's fat."

My world collapsed as his words rang in my ears. *I'm fat?* I wondered in confusion.

How am I fat?

Up until that point, *fat* was never a word used to describe me. I was intelligent. I was athletic. I was nice. I was the girl that all the neighborhood boys lined up to race, and—always under the watchful eye of my mother posted on our front steps—I would leave them in the dust. I was a "guys' girl," I related to the boys more than the girls. But I was not fat.

How could TJ think I'm fat?

All school year, I had gone out of my way to catch his attention. I made sure to laugh at all his jokes, even when they were corny. I frequently positioned myself around him to make sure he could see me. Just moments ago, he had flirted with me by slapping the back of my thigh. How could he not like me?

In no time, my day went from amazing to horrible. The possibility of TJ and me being together nose-dived with his rejection, and that experience would set the precedent for how I would feel for the rest of my life. Suddenly, and without warning, I was the ugly, fat girl.

In 1996, growing up in the inner city of Cleveland, Ohio, I was often lonely. I wasn't an only child but because my sister who was nine years older had cerebral palsy, I didn't have a consistent playmate.

My mom was super strict and there was no way I could go over anybody's house, play in their backyard, or even outside of her line of vision. The only thing I had were those legendary neighborhood races on the weekends. They were a huge source of self-esteem since none of the boys could beat me. I was the only girl, and boys would line up to race, but outside of that, I was homebound.

On Sundays, there was at least some social interaction at church with other kids. My mom was big on church, so we went every weekend. As a result, I received foundational Biblical teachings. I was also able to develop a personal relationship with God outside of the weekend services. I was always praying or talking to God as a child and never felt like I couldn't go to Him about anything.

During the week, every day at 5:30 am on the dot my mom

woke me and my sister up with breakfast ready. She was huge on structure and routine so there wasn't a school day that went by when this didn't happen.

"Eat your oatmeal, it will keep you full," she would tell us.

Mom was big on us staying full because she was a single parent doing it all and the only breadwinner. My grandmother was also in the household; however, she was diagnosed with Schizophrenia. Whether she would be emotionally, mentally, or physically available to assist with parenting depended on whether her medications were the right dosage or if she was even taking them at all.

Back when walking in the hood was safe, I walked to school every morning. If my grandmother was with me and wasn't doing well, she could be caught having a conversation with a nearby pole. Or, one with just herself. There were days I would sneak out of the house without her and walk myself to school rather than have to snap her out of one of those states and help *her* walk *me* to school. Those moments when she was with me could be so embarrassing.

On my way to school, there was a corner store just off East 150th St. and Harvard Ave. They had the best selection of $.05 candy, $.25 bag of chips, and $.25 pops and juices. These were my morning snacks that I used my $1.00 lunch money to purchase. It was never a question that I wouldn't get my morning snacks because everybody in my neighborhood did. Having snacks was a sign that you were cool. As a result, I developed a routine of snacking that stemmed from the culture in my community.

If I made it to school early enough, I was able to eat breakfast… again. I just loved those peanut butter and jelly graham crackers and breakfast donuts! On a good day, I would have eaten three times in a matter of hours by the time the school day began. After my third breakfast, I was already looking forward to lunch. Then, after school, it was time to hit the corner store on the way home to get my afternoon snack, which, of course, was another bag of chips, a can of pop or juice, and more candy.

Now, even though I was told by my mother *not* to go to the store, I didn't have any supervision, so who was going to stop me? I was on all accounts a latch-key kid, and from the time I got home, I was on my own for a whole two hours. I would let my sister in when she got home from high school and knew not to open the door to strangers.

After school, my sister and grandmother were doing their own thing, so the TV was my babysitter and food was my friend. I frequently turned to food out of loneliness and boredom. In the mornings, since my mother would have already left for work, I was responsible for getting to school on time. I knew that if I caught the entire episode of my favorite show, "Sailor Moon," I was running late. A lot of kids around me were responsible for their own well-being, so this wasn't a big deal.

In our neighborhood, my house was a dream. My mom had a stable job and was a manager at an insurance agency. At age 33, she was considered an "older mom" and wore suits every single day. We had breakfast every day at the same time and dinner too. All of our physical needs were taken care of and then some. I knew that even though we lived in the hood, we didn't have it nearly as bad as my neighbors who I could hear screaming at night or whose parents were strung out on drugs. We didn't take family vacations, but my life was a charm in comparison. The darker side of our home had been removed when my mom finally kicked my dad out.

Back in the day, my dad was a huge drug lord in the city and probably one of the main sources for the decline of the east side of Cleveland. Typically dressed in furs, alligator shoes, and leathered down from head to toe, he was the classic depiction of a kingpin. Crack was his business, and the people in our community were his clients. In addition to his drug-selling, he was a drug user *and* a domestic abuser. My mom ended up in the hospital too many times from broken jaws and beatings, but my sister has the lifelong evidence of my father's nasty temper. One time, while my sister was a baby, he was home alone with her and got so sick of her crying that he threw her against the garage. She was six months old. That incident caused her to develop cerebral palsy. She has been walking with a limp and dragging her foot ever since she learned to walk. Finally, my mom had enough and kicked my dad out. I remember the day he left like it was yesterday. He kissed me on the cheek, and I never saw him again. I was two years old.

I never consciously missed my dad, but in retrospect, I do think having a house full of women caused me to overemphasize attention from males at a young age. At just seven years old, I let someone else's perception flip my world upside down. Little TJ did a number on me with his comment about my weight, and his words planted a seed of discontentment with my body. I went home that day and squinted at my reflection in the mirror, trying to figure out what made someone fat. The only point of reference I had at the time were TV characters. Characters like Uncle Phil from "The Fresh Prince of Bel-Air" and Carl Winslow from "Family Matters" seemed to be "heavy" to me. But I wasn't as big as them, so I was still confused. Then there was my role model Brandy from the hit show *Moesha*. People loved to tell me how much I looked like Brandy, and I loved every time I received the compliment. I was good for rocking my braids just like she did and aimed my style after hers. Moesha always got the popular guy on TV and had a group of friends surrounding her. She was intelligent and everybody liked her. As much as people said I looked like someone who was pretty and thin, how could I then be fat? I was not the Kim, Moesha's best friend who was plus-sized. I was the Moesha. Period!

Chapter 1

As I analyzed the 7-year-old image reflecting in the mirror and compared it to all these TV characters, I didn't understand how someone else saw me as fat, but I did become aware that *something* was wrong. And after that day, I became bent on figuring out how to fix myself so that others would accept me.

Chapter 2
FIELD DAY

Being popular in school was always a good look in the movies and TV shows that kept me company after school. So, when TJ's comment cemented my low-ranking social status, I struggled with how I could climb the ranks. It seemed that even though I came from a good home, had the best clothes, and was smart and athletic, these attributes weren't enough. Could it be that my cute, pleated name-brand skirts were overshadowed by my mom's no-nonsense business attire whenever she appeared at my school? The popular girls' moms were the fly girls dressed in trendy, stylish outfits that were youthful and fun. I had naturally adopted a more mature disposition from my rigorous, studious home environment, but noticed that the popular girls' spirited personalities were drawing boys like bees to honey. Yeah, I was the girl next door. The girl who boys were friends with. The girl they could race on the street and wrestle with. But I wanted to be the one the boys desired. I wanted to be popular. Also working against me socially was that I was the girl whose sister dragged her foot and whose grandmother talked to herself publicly. What I finally settled on was

Chapter 2

that while I couldn't change who I was related to, I could change how I came off to others. I could change me.

I started working overtime to fit in with the very girls who had whispered behind my back, talking stuff to TJ. I would be extra friendly to them and go out of my way to hang out with them, but my attempts weren't as successful as I wanted them to be. Because I was naturally more of a "guys' girl" and couldn't help but feel more comfortable with the boys, kicking it with the girls didn't last long.

By third grade, I may not have had the boys' romantic interest, but I did have their respect. I was still thriving in my athletic element, and my impressive speed, power, and agility became my foundation for confidence. I could always find security in being a champion. But the day came when even that was challenged. I was at school, and it was Field Day. Field Day is every student athlete's dream. It's when you get to show off and excel in every fun game the school offers. This particular day, we were playing kickball, and when it was my turn to kick, all the guys on the opposing team started screaming, "Go out! Go out!" That was a huge compliment because it meant I could kick far. If you were a poor kicker they would scream the opposite, "Come in! Come in!" which was blatant disrespect. I took my turn and did not disappoint. The ball soared, and I headed for first base. When I got there, full of adrenaline and pride at my achievement, my victory was immediately dashed by the girl manning first base. "You only kicked far because you got big legs," she snarled. "You the same size as the boys." I looked down at my legs, but instead of seeing my legs, I saw my belly falling over the waistline of my shorts. Not only did I have big legs but apparently, I had a big stomach too. My feelings plummeted. No matter what I did to earn the approval of my peers, I couldn't seem to make them forget the one thing I couldn't control: my weight.

On the home front, my mom's message to me was the opposite. "You're not fat, you're solid," she would chant. But you know how kids learn more by what is caught not taught? My mom would drill into my head over and over that my size was fine but would struggle with her own weight gain. Naturally a petite woman, she rocked a size four most of her life, so when she suddenly shot up to a size eight, she acted like the world was ending. "I can't wear my suits!" she cried in fear, and I witnessed firsthand the emotional effects of a slowed-down metabolism most women experience in their 30s. Around third grade I watched her struggle with her weight. This showed me that being bigger was not a good thing. It also taught me that even when in my eyes my mom looked fine, in her self-view, something was wrong.

I adopted that same self-view. And though initially I didn't think I was overweight, I started peering in the mirror and wondering, "Do I look fat in these jeans?" Here I was, a child sharing the inner thoughts of 30-year-old women.

By fourth grade, mom remarried to my stepdad who was a minister and a good guy. He had a son and daughter who visited every weekend. It was the first time I had playmates in the home, and it was so much fun. But it was also another opportunity to start seeing how I didn't seem to measure up in the looks department. My stepsister was another fair-skinned, long hair, petite type, and my cousin-in-law was too. One Easter Sunday, we got dressed in our puffy pink dresses. Photo-ready, we ended up at my stepdad's family's house. The only problem was when they took the photo with the old-school Polaroid that made you wait for the result even after waving the picture in the air, the outcome wasn't what I was expecting. Instead of seeing three beautiful girls matching in their pink Easter Sunday bests, I saw two gorgeous lighter-skinned, thin-lipped girls, and one big chocolate girl right in the middle. It wasn't just that I didn't look like my friends. It was that, in my eyes, I looked worse than them.

Chapter 2

"My lips are too big!" I would tell my mom. "My nose is too wide!" I wanted a nose and lips like my stepsister and cousin-in-law. Even my sister had smaller lips than I did. "You're beautiful!" My mom would argue back. "You're going to love your lips when you grow up!" But I couldn't see it. All I saw was how different I looked, and all I could focus on was how much bigger I was than them. On top of my size, my hair was kinkier. My mom would press the hell out of my 4C coils. She was constantly trying to big me up. "You're so pretty!" she would say. "You have beautiful eyes." But I didn't care. I wanted to look like the girls who got TJ's attention. Even when I was in my neighborhood with my cousin and stepsister, I saw how boys showered them with attention in a way they never did with me. They were flirted with, and I was tolerated. I was just one of the guys.

In fifth grade, things took a drastic turn when my mom announced that we were moving. My mom and stepdad had been married about a year and half when they claimed that we were getting a bigger house. "Y'all are going to love it!" they said, making it seem like we were on the come-up. This was a pivotal time for me because fifth grade was the start of my middle school years. I would be entering into a new stage of academia which meant the cool factor would be even more important. On the one hand, I grew excited about the prospect of a fresh start with a new move. I could finally be the popular girl! On the other hand, I had acquired a level of respect in my old neighborhood. I was the smart, bubbly, athletic girl. Maybe I wasn't as popular as I wanted to be, but everyone knew me. I was safe. I was also a little disappointed I wasn't going to attend the middle school in my old neighborhood which was still a good school in the inner city. It was so good you had to be tested in, which I had been. Ultimately, I settled on the view that this move was my chance to be the one the boys wanted and the one the girls wanted to be. We were moving to Maple Heights, a more suburban neighborhood back then that was still mixed with white folks.

One of our first orders of business was for me to get a physical before the school year started. My pediatrician weighed me and announced my weight in the small hospital room. "150 pounds!" he said.

I gulped as the words echoed in my mind. *150 pounds? Is that a lot?*

"Just make sure you watch what she's eating," my doctor told my mom. I was 10 years old and not more than 5' 3". "Mom, is 150 pounds a lot?" I asked not too long after my appointment with the doctor. But my mom was quick to respond, "You're just solid, that's all," she stated. "You're *not* fat."

At that point, I had a number that seemed like it validated what others had been saying about me, but I still had conflicting views on what that number meant. The doctor said it meant my mom needed to watch what I was eating, but my mom kept saying it didn't mean I was fat. It wasn't until a friend and I shared our weights with each other that I had evidence of what I'd been suspecting. "You weigh 150 pounds?" my friend asked me, and I nodded. "I weigh 97 pounds," she revealed. My jaw nearly dropped. My friend was almost half my size, and we were the same age! How could 150 pounds *not* be big if it was almost *double* the weight of my friend? That was a moment that solidified to me that regardless of *what* my mother kept telling me, I was *definitely* fat. But even with this new knowledge, I held high hopes for my new beginning. I didn't care what the scale said, I was still going to be a fly girl. I was still going to be Moesha.

For my first day of school, my mom made sure my hair was done in latch hooks, a style of wavy braids that Brandy wore and that was popular with a lot of girls back in the day. I was so excited about my first day, that I spent the whole night before picking out my outfit. I settled on a blue bodysuit that I stole from my sister's closet, baggy high-waisted jeans, and a black-rimmed hat in honor of Moesha. Now, the fact that I was able to wear my sister's clothes even though I was nine years younger lets you know I was a big girl. But that wasn't what I chose to focus on. Instead, my head was swimming with excitement for my new life. I would have boys. I would have friends. I would have it all. The next day, I eagerly went to school in my cute fit. Confidently, I walked the halls that led to my classroom. This was my moment of popularity! My eyes sparkled with hope and lit up even more when I saw the boys in my class awaiting my arrival. They had been told they were getting a new girl. But upon entering, my high hopes crashed. The boys took one look at me, smacked their teeth, huffed, and rolled their eyes. "She's ugly" they spat. "She's fat." My heart was broken. I wanted to run out and cry. Once again, my looks were a letdown. Once again, the boys didn't want me. Once again, I was the fat girl.

Chapter 3
MEAN GIRLS

Middle school was a nightmare, plain and simple. Not only did the boys not like me, but our supposed bigger, more amazing dream house was outdated, and my room was in the cold, dreary attic. It was always freezing in that attic, and I hated it. Our old house had been newly renovated, and we had so many childhood memories there. We were happy there. I have no idea how my mom thought this new house was better. It was clear she and my stepdad had sold us kids a pipe dream. And then, all of a sudden, my stepbrother and sister stopped coming over every weekend because my mom was upset about them visiting so much. As a result, I was back to playing alone.

Academically, my new school system was behind, and they were covering stuff in my fifth-grade year that I had already learned in third grade. Because my mom had never let me go to the more disadvantaged inner-city schools and only kept me in the charter school, I was more advanced than even the suburban school in Maple Heights. Since my classes were redundant, I knew all the answers, so when the teacher asked the question, I, of course, raised my hand with the right response. This put me in the "know-it-all" category, and the other kids teased me for it. "She thinks she's so smart!" they sneered. That followed me for the rest of the school year. I started questioning myself. *Should I have raised my hand? Maybe I'll just sit here and say nothing at all.* It was the first time I felt like I needed to dim my light.

My very first day of middle school, I faced the cafeteria challenge. You know when you're trying to figure out who to sit with at lunch? Lucky for me the popular girls invited me to their table. One girl was heavy-chested and dating the most popular boy in school. Another girl was light-skinned, skinny, and dating the second most popular boy. The other two girls were their lackeys who followed them around everywhere. The girls started vetting me to see if I could hang with them. "Where are you from? Who did your hair? What are you wearing?" They were really into labels and wanted to know about my clothing brands. Then some boys came by and started making beats on the table. The girls started dancing and invited me to join, but I stayed in my seat. At the time, I didn't know how to dance and was too insecure. After lunch, we went out for recess, and the girls went behind nearby trailers on the school property and started twerking. I was in shock. I had been super sheltered and had never even seen twerking before. At that time, I was still very much a kid, and dancing like that was intimidating. Later that evening at home, when my mom asked how the first day went, I said "ok," but spent the whole night over-analyzing my every move and the initial negative response from the boys. *Did I do enough to impress the popular girls? Was it my outfit that made the boys not like me? Why did they think I was fat?*

The next day at lunch, the popular girls said I couldn't sit with them. They were the meanest of the mean girls, and I was crushed. I ended up sitting by myself at lunch for the rest of the year. That year was so hard. I went from being someone everyone knew, liked, and respected in my old neighborhood to being the know-it-all no one wanted to be friends with. I constantly felt rejected, out of place, ugly, and, of course, *fat*. None of the boys liked me, and I dictated my worth based on their interest. Or lack thereof. I couldn't be further away from my idol, Moesha, if I had tried.

My loneliness and depression from my popularity being at rock bottom led me to do what I always did. I turned to food. Even when we moved, my daily schedule still revolved around eating and food was my primary means for passing the time. I just loved me some oatmeal cream pies! Of course, I ate the generic ones because my mom wasn't about to pay extra money for the name brand. Pair one with a tall glass of Dairyman's red juice or pink lemonade, and I was in heaven! We were big juice drinkers in our home. No water allowed. That was the culture I was raised in, and that was the culture I carried into our new residence. My mom wasn't as much of a foodie as me and my sister, but her desire to show us love carried into not having limits on what we were eating. Often, parents want to give their children what they didn't have growing up. Letting us overeat was a response to the lack she faced in her childhood.

In urban communities, it's typical to face food deserts. There's a convenience store on every corner filled with high-cholesterol, sugary, processed foods, yet very few grocery stores nearby offering healthier food or fresh produce. You have to go *out* of the hood to get to those spaces, and it's obvious the intent is to keep impoverished communities impoverished. Our mental health is connected to our physical health, and what we put into our bodies affects our levels of depression and anxiety. Then people of color get addicted to the unhealthy lifestyle and find ourselves in cycles of addiction. That's where I was at just 10 years old. I was addicted to unhealthy food because I didn't know any better. I imitated those around me and wouldn't be able to break the cycle for a very long time.

According to the National Library of Medicine (https://pmc.ncbi.nlm.nih.gov/articles/PMC7852671/), studies show that processed sugar is just as addictive as illegal drugs such as cocaine, yet sugar is perfectly legal and included in many of the foods Americans eat regularly. In lower socio-economic communities, the options are slim to find convenient, nutritious items, and it's rare for those living in these spaces to adopt a healthy lifestyle. No one taught us about portion control or sugar consumption growing up in the hood. I would come home every day and prepare whatever snack satisfied my sugar cravings without a second thought. My mom would buy a box of orange creamsicles, and I would kill the whole box all by myself in a day. Every day after school, I would go home, watch my stories like "Days of Our Lives" and "Passions," and eat my snack before mom arrived for dinner. During this time, I was feeding off of unhealthy ideas about love and relationships as well as food. TV was my constant escape from reality along with my snacks.

In the summer, my eating habits were worse because I was home all day. On summer vacation, I would cook chili dogs for the house and smash five of them all on my own! At noon, when Sesame Street came on, I knew it was snack time, so I'd start in on some Twinkies. By the end of the day, the whole box would be gone. I lived for food simply because there was nothing else to do. My brain began connecting food with my daily routine, which often revolved around different television shows I watched. So, even though *I* couldn't see the extra weight I was carrying until others brought it to my attention, it's understandable that others could. Eating all day like that you can't help but put on a few pounds!

Inspired by movies I watched, I decided over the summer that when the new year began, I would become the bully. Just like those who had previously rejected me, I would become a mean girl. Since I couldn't change my weight to combat the stigma of being the unpopular fat girl, I would change my personality.

The first day of sixth grade, I sauntered in in jeans, a pink shirt, and glitter lotion. My hair was laid, relaxed, and in flat twists sprinkled with butterfly clips just like Brittany Spears used to wear. *I'm popular now!* I thought, confident and eager for a fresh start. And guess what? I did become popular, just like I wanted. Unfortunately, I had to go out of my way to be an awful human being to achieve it. I was quick to give my teachers a hard time, disrupting the class to make inappropriate jokes so the other students would laugh. Detentions and phone calls at home to my mom started flooding in. The teachers hated me but the kids loved it. Suddenly, I had friends. I started dressing just like the popular girls in my pink velour jumpsuit. After Christmas kids always wanted to see who had new fits and I was eager to show off mine to my new friends. Boys began paying attention to me.

Being a mean girl is working for me! I thought, so I kept at it. Until one day I was a mean girl to the wrong girl.

This particular day, I was picking on a girl at school while outside at recess. I targeted her because we had the same issues. She was overweight with acne and was brand new to the school. Since I was insecure with my weight and appearance, I figured she was too and thought she would be easy pickings. But she warned me, "Leave me alone or we gone' fight." By then, there was a group swarming us, and since I was more popular, they were on my side, egging me on. They had my back. Or so I thought. I was high off the attention and cocky, so I went in on her verbally. Before I knew it, we were going at it physically, but, to my surprise, I lost the fight. It was my very first real fight. Before then, I had only play-wrestled with boys and didn't know what I was getting myself into. What made things worse was that in the middle of the fight, I started screaming, "I'll kill you!"

Chapter 3

That landed me in the expulsion zone. My mom, stepdad and I had to go in front of the school board to plead my case as to why I shouldn't be expelled. My parents fought for me, telling the school I had a clean record before then and this was a one-time offense. Thankfully, I got off on a two-week suspension on top of having to write an apology letter to the girl I fought and the school board.

At home, my mom was not one to play. I had the worst time off ever. A very religious woman, she made me write the whole book of Proverbs and Revelations from the Bible from top to bottom on top of hand-written book reports. There was absolutely no TV for two whole weeks. It was hell. When I got back to school, the reality of my loss was clear in the students' attitudes toward me. After that fight, I lost all of my so-called friends. No one acknowledged or even talked to me when I returned from suspension. I was once again alone.

Even though it was a hard lesson, I learned from that experience that some people will only be on your side when it seems it will benefit *them*. The kids I thought were my friends never really were. They were just sailing on the coattails of my fleeting popularity. After that fight, the rest of the school year, I flew under the radar. My grades were ok, but I was back to coping with loneliness through food.

By seventh grade, my appearance was challenged even more by a bad case of acne. Now I *really* didn't want to be seen. I tried to be invisible by minimizing myself and sitting in the back of the classroom. I stopped raising my hand or answering questions and rarely talked to anyone. I didn't want anyone to know I existed. Where I had been a math genius before, by seventh grade, I fell behind academically. Stuff just wasn't clicking anymore, and I couldn't keep up with the lessons. Around that time, unbeknownst to me, my ADHD had kicked in, and it was hard for me to pay attention and focus. Even when my mom would take me to the library and I would check out books, I couldn't get past the third page due to my short attention span, so I'd rent DVDs instead.

During these years, I spent a lot of time sitting in class daydreaming about the life I *wanted* to live. The life I saw others living in movies and on TV shows. Then I developed another big crush. Tommy. Tommy was light-skinned with long curly hair decked in a classic 90s-oversized white-T and Girbaud jeans. The nice thing about Tommy was that he wasn't obnoxious like the other popular boys. He was actually friendly and kept to himself a lot. I knew his cousin because we attended the same church, so we had kind of grown up together from a distance. Once in a while, Tommy would talk to me, but only as a friend. Then Sweetest Day came. In middle school, the school sold $1 carnations to the students to buy for their crush as a fundraiser. Ugh, I hated those days! Those school events were so isolating for certain people. I was never the girl who received a carnation which added to my already poor self-esteem. There were the girls who got one or two, and then there were the girls like Amber who had like twelve! Amber was short and cute with long hair. She was friendly and never mean, but the day she received a carnation from Tommy, I felt some kind of way about her. Then they started dating and my dreams of him and I being together went down the drain.

My self-esteem reached an all-time low during seventh grade, and nothing changed in eighth. Food was my only constant companion. I just loved going to the all-you-can-eat buffet at Hometown Buffet on Sundays after church and loading my plate with only desserts. Even though I was still athletic, I no longer had an outlet, so the pounds just piled on. My plans to join organized sports in my old neighborhood were sabotaged by adjusting to the new school environment in Maple Heights and not feeling like I fit in anywhere. No matter how hard I tried, I just wasn't accepted. To cope, I binged on '90s rom-coms. I saw the ugly duckling-turned-swan in *16 Candles* and *Pretty in Pink* and waited for that moment in my own life.

Then, finally, my moment arrived. Ninth grade hit. And I became a *fly girl*.

Chapter 4
FLY GIRL

At the end of my eighth grade year, I made a really good friend named Channon. Channon was the typical girl next door, easygoing, and the boys loved her. She was pretty with chocolate brown skin, funny, and even though she got along with the popular girls, was still super approachable. Channon was the extrovert to my introvert and let me kick it with her about a month prior to eighth-grade ending. Once we graduated from eighth grade, she became my first best friend to actually make it through the summer.

That summer, we walked everywhere, and without me knowing it, the weight started falling off. That was back when you left the house at 10 am and didn't come back home 'till 7 pm. Thank God my mother had finally loosened the reins and was giving me more freedom. Channon and I would go to her grandmother's house where she would teach me how to dance and her grandmother would cook for us, or we would visit her different friends' houses. Because *she* accepted me, Channon's friends did too. That summer, my popularity status started climbing, my body was changing, and by the end of the summer, I was eager to step into my new position as a fly girl.

Two weeks before school started, Mom took me to Kaufmann's (now Macy's) and I tried on a Marc Jacobs Echo red hoodie dress. "Ariel, do you know that dress is a size double zero?" my mom said, staring at the tag in shock. "Ok," I said. I had no idea what that even meant, but I knew it meant something by the look she gave me. For some reason, that whole summer, I never noticed that my clothes were fitting differently, looser. It wasn't until we went shopping for the new school year that it was brought to my attention that I was suddenly a double zero.

To complement my new clothes, I asked Mom if I could ditch my micro braids and get my hair relaxed. For years my mother would tell me how long and beautiful my hair was, but because of my own insecurities, I never believed her. The boys back then used to claim that girls who wore braids and weaves were bald-headed, and it was a running joke in middle school that I must be bald because I always wore braids. So, in spite of my mom's *constant* affirmations, that's what I believed. Even though my mom would also always hype me up about my full lips and slanted "Chinese" eyes, I was a victim of the messaging of colorism that aired in most of the 1990s TV shows. Normally the female-character-lead was light-skinned, skinny, with long hair, while her sidekick was darker-complected. Think Gina and Pam from "Martin". Whether it was TV, music videos, or rap songs, women have historically been objectified by men based on our skin tone, hair type, and body shape. Young girls like me grew up *only* seeing beauty in *one* form, and many felt deficient if we didn't fit into *that* form. My skin tone is actually more of a medium brown, but because it wasn't light, I was thrown into the category of being dark-skinned. As a result of constant belittling from my peers and the colorist messaging on television, body dysmorphia, and imposter syndrome became a real struggle for me. Even as an adult, I still battle to see myself as I truly am.

At my request, my mom gave me money to go to the local salon before ninth grade started. When I got that perm, my hair dropped down to the middle of my back. I couldn't believe it! I looked in the mirror and whipped it from side to side. I was stunned. My stylist raved, "Girl, you have long, healthy hair!" and for the first time, I could see it.

The first day of ninth grade, I walked in wearing a white crop top with a sheer back, fitted light-blue jeans, and fake Steve Madden Manolo Blahnik shoes from Kaufman's. Sitting in homeroom, the boyfriend of the most popular girl from fifth grade touched the back of my bra strap. "Ariel?" he said in surprise. I turned around to look at him. "Wow. You look—different." Four years after the beginning of middle school, the most popular boy from back then gives me this compliment. He was a part of the same crew of boys that would ignore me and tease me. His compliment was the start of it all. There was no doubt about it. I was fly.

It was still warm outside, and me and my girl Channon were still walking. After school, we would end up at the park and watch the boys play basketball, or we would head to the stadium or corner store to chill, and the boys would be there. All of a sudden, boys started asking for my number. Channon had always gotten the attention, but now, they were after me. One day, I started collecting boys' numbers, and at the end of the evening, Channon had me tally up how many numbers I had. After I ruffled through the little strips of papers, I was in shock. There were 23 boys' phone numbers in my hands. Channon was like, "Girl, you got a lot of dudes!" To make matters worse, I had a little Nokia cell phone. You couldn't tell me nothing. I was talking to all kinds of boys. I thought I was the sh*t. Around this time, Tommy, my crush from sixth grade, was in one of my classes and saw me. He put his hand on my leg and said, "Damn, Ariel, you skinny as 'F!'" I was thinking, *finally*!

The first week of school, there were all kinds of celebrations. We had homecoming week which included a bonfire all week, and all types of activities to be social with the other students. Homecoming night, on my way to the bonfire, a guy named D approached me. Smoothly he said, "You should call me," then gave me his number. I took it and agreed. I ended up talking to four more boys as Channon and I walked to the bonfire in Stafford Park, and I had forgotten all about D. This was back when people would ghost ride their whips, and the senior boys flossed their 32-inch rims, blaring their sounds. The classics (the old school cars boys flaunted back then) were big, the flag girls were goin', and the band was fire. It was wild. It was the first time I felt good about myself. I had a good friend. I was getting compliments. Everybody was feeling me. My outfits were poppin' because my mom had finally let me start picking out my own clothes. And most importantly, my body was thin.

Soon after me and Channon made it to the bleachers and started dancing, I felt a tug on my shoulder. I looked over and it was D, but I squinted my eyes, trying to place him. "Oh, you don't remember me?" he said playfully. "I just gave you my number." I smiled slowly. "Oh, yeah." D was a straight hood dude. Caramel skin, baggy clothes, and eyes always low from being high. You could smell the weed before you ever saw him coming. He was every mother's nightmare and definitely not someone *my* mother would have approved of. I don't know what it was about him that attracted me most out of all the boys I was talking to. He wasn't that cute, average height, and walked with some kind of limp where he leaned and dragged his foot. Apparently, he had gotten into a fight in juvi and had been walking like that ever since. I think I was compassionate about it because of my sister's limp and from being in a household where my relatives had ailments that others would make fun of. Maybe I also fell for him because D made me laugh.

D invited me to his house the next day and made me a sandwich and noodles. It might as well have been steak and lobster as far as I was concerned! I thought that was everything. When he went to cook, there were some burnt corn dogs still in the oven, and he said, "I don't know who made that, but they need to try again." That made me laugh so hard. I stuck with him for two years over that. Outside of D's sense of humor and cooking for me, I had no other qualities of what to look for in a dating partner. Even though my stepdad was in the picture, I never had a "daddy-daughter" relationship with him that could teach me value from a man's perspective. My mom was very protective over me, and my stepdad and I never spent time alone. I never had a father-figure and, as a result, made poor choices for a long time when it came to relationships.

During ninth grade, my eating habits had diminished significantly because I wasn't sitting around the house all day watching TV. I was walking with Channon and then started kicking it with D. My mom would give me $5, and sometimes I would split a $5 footlong with Channon and that would be the only thing I ate after school. No more chips, candy, and pop. No more eating three breakfasts in the morning. The positive was that I wasn't overeating and using food as a coping mechanism. The negative was that I was undereating and not getting enough nutrition. On top of my undereating, I was constantly burning calories walking. I soon started burning calories with sex.

D had been pressuring me for sex for about two weeks before I caved. He was 16 and I was 14. I had barely kissed a guy. I only talked to the boys I was getting numbers from. I had never met up with any of them in person or done anything physical with them. I had just learned how to twerk! D was out of my league with experience, but I was afraid to lose him, so I gave in. My other friends were already sexually active, so my culture was once again influencing me.

My very first time skipping school, me, D, Channon, and her boyfriend all kicked it at my house. Me and D were upstairs, and Channon and her guy were downstairs, but we had an extra companion in the mix. D's brother, who was 19 and known to be a shady character, had popped up with D. While me and D were doing our thing and Channon and her man were doing theirs, D's brother was roaming the house. A week later, my mom's house got broken into. Two of the robbers held my grandmother hostage while the other one stole over $5,000 worth of my stepbrother's video games and technology from the basement. My brother had all the latest like PlayStation, Nintendo, and Xbox as well as all name-brand gear that he had paid for with his job as a golf caddy. When he was 12, my brother moved in with us after he started getting into trouble at his mom's house. When the robbery happened, I was shocked, scared, and knew it had to be D's brother. That meant D was in on it too.

In the police report, my family and I had to say who had been in the house around that time, and I had to admit that D, Channon, her dude, and D's brother were there. "Why were these boys in the house? Were y'all havin' sex?" my mom demanded incredulously. I lowered my gaze, scrunched my shoulders, and nodded. Of course, she was livid. I was immediately on lockdown. I couldn't go anywhere but church and home every day for the rest of ninth grade. She took away my phone and forced me to write the whole book of Proverbs for 90 days. Channon's mom was notified and she cut off our friendship since Channon was having sex at my house and she blamed me for being the bad influence. It also came out that Channon's boyfriend was older than her, so her mom filed statutory rape charges. Our friendship was over after that. In no time, I had lost my virginity, my boyfriend, and my best friend.

Channon's boyfriend had a sister, and when she found out about the rape charges, she blamed it on me. About a week after the robbery, while I was walking home from school, the sister jumped me along with four of her friends in front of my house. These girls were all friends with Channon, but instead of being upset with her, they took it out on me. Thankfully, I didn't have any real injuries, but the damage to my self-esteem was huge. I had finally made it into the popular clique and, within a span of a week, it was over. These were girls I thought I was cool with, but they took everything out on me and stayed friends with Channon, even though *her* mother was the one who pressed charges.

You would think after all that I would have broken up with D, but about a month later, I snuck out and went to his house. That's when I saw his brother rocking one of *my* brother's sweaters. It was way too big and swallowed his small frame. The evidence was clear as day that he had robbed us. I didn't say anything though. I still kept messing with D. At that point, he was my only companion. No one else would talk to me. Just like in middle school, after I lost that fight, no one wanted anything to do with me after I got jumped.

I was being risky though, sneaking and seeing D, and eventually, my mom found out. She caught me about to walk up to his house and pulled up on me in her car. "Oh, you want to disrespect me?" She yelled. "Square up if you think you grown!" I yelled back but still got in the car. When we got back home, she went upstairs to put on her Timberlands. I would never touch my mother so that altercation was basically her popping me a few times and stumping me. After that, I was back on punishment and forced to write the whole book of Proverbs. There was no TV. No phone. It was hell, but I was so stuck on D that I kept sneaking out. That whole time period I would sneak out, get caught, and get put back on punishment.

Chapter 4

The day came when D ended up going to jail for robbery. Afterward, he was sent to juvenile hall for eight long months for violating his parole. The day he told me, I was at his house kicking it with his sister and she handed me the phone. I was in disbelief at the news that he would be out of my life for so long. The reason D had gotten so much time was because he had numerous charges on his record. He had been stealing from houses all around Maple Heights, and everybody at school knew it. People would come up to me, "Yo boyfriend locked up for hittin' licks!" But I would shake my head. I didn't want to believe that this wasn't just a one off. The truth was he had been committing robberies even while we were talking on the phone to each other. I would ask what he was doing, and he would say, "Oh, I'm just out chillin'," but then I would hear him running and breathing hard. I had been so sheltered that I wasn't street-savvy enough to realize he was a liar and a thief. I was so sprung that sometimes, that $5 my mom gave me for lunch would go to him when he came at me with some sob story about needing to buy clothes for job interviews. I would hand over all the money on me and go without lunch all week. But as toxic as he was in my life, D was my closest friend. Without him, I fell into depression. Once again, I was alone and unpopular. This time instead of overeating, heartbreak made my eating habits pretty much nonexistent. Heartbreak is the best diet pill for me and my body stayed thin. I put my hair back into braids and went back into my shell. My stint of popularity had crashed after only two months.

But what I've learned is that when God doesn't want me somewhere, He will pull me out quick. I had gotten a little attention, and I started wildin' out. I ditched all of my home-taught values and started living fast. But I wasn't called to that life. I was different. Unfortunately, I wouldn't see it this way for many years.

At the time, all I knew was that I wanted acceptance. I wanted friendship. I wanted love. And it was all gone. That's when I started skipping school. I hated going to school because I had no one to talk to. This behavior followed me into tenth grade. I would either walk around or go back home when I was supposed to be at school. I went from being a straight-A student to failing. My mom finally got fed up. "You gone' have to do something, Ariel!" she told me.

That's when I started running track. And running track changed my life.

Chapter 5
TRACK STAR

In tenth-grade homeroom, I got cool with a quiet, soft-spoken girl named Tracy. We would have small banter, which, at the time, was the highlight of my social life. She was nice, and I needed nice. In homeroom one day, Tracy asked if I could kick it after school, but I told her I wasn't allowed. I was still on lockdown after all my shenanigans with D. But then she said, "I run track. You should try out for the track team." Memories of me racing the boys in my old neighborhood flashed through my mind. *I used to beat them,* I thought with a rush of excitement. *Let me see if my mom will let me do it.* I figured I would give it a shot, even though I doubted she would be on it. To my surprise, when I asked her that evening, Mom said yes. I tried out and made varsity as a sophomore. I was good. Really good.

Before practice, I was stretching with Tracy, who was a hurdler, when I heard the coach say to me, "Baker, go with the hurdlers!" I didn't even know what hurdling was, but when I got on the field, I killed it. I ended up doing 100-meter hurdles, the 4x1, long jump, *and* pole vaulting. The senior girls who were at the top of their game were leaving out, so the track team was reinventing itself. That meant there was room for newbies like me at the top. Even though I was new, I was keeping up with Tracy, who had been running for years. I had no prior history of organized sports or running other than those races I did as a kid, but I was a natural. I started practicing and conditioning like crazy, and, as a result, my body began putting on muscle. I even had abs! My eating habits were better too because I had a reason to eat better. My coaches started barking that we needed to eat for energy so that we could win. My mindset around food became that food was fuel for my body to win races and become a state qualifier. Complex carbs were viewed as a good thing because pasta and rice would last long enough to burn in meets and result in optimum performance. This was a huge switch because now I was eating to meet a short-term goal, instead of eating out of boredom to pass the time.

I started swapping out my chicken nuggets for salads at lunch, and my mom was getting on board with making healthier meals once she saw my change. She would pack protein bars and exchange the Toaster Strudels and Pop-Tarts for oatmeal with fruit, hard-boiled eggs, or anything that would be healthier, high in fiber, and fast for me to eat. "Ariel, I know you have practice today, so I got you a salad with tuna on it," Mom would say. "Ariel, I got these Carnation shakes for you for when you don't have time to make breakfast!" she piped. My mom was all in when it came to supporting my new diet and lifestyle and I began using those quick snacks in the mornings. I needed them because I was constantly running late to school since I was more independent now and mom wasn't waking me up. I was also catching rides with friends instead of taking the bus. This social change added to my diet change as well. Food had always been my friend, but in high school, I had real friends. I didn't need food in the way I used to, and it was no longer my focal point.

Track instilled discipline in me in so many areas. I had previously been failing ninth grade, but I had to keep up my grades to stay on the team in tenth. It also helped that I had no access to D, so I had stopped skipping school. When D went to jail, it saved me. I had no other choice but to focus on classes. The teachers went from not seeing me to seeing me, and some didn't even recognize me. They were like, "Who are you again?" I had even picked up some extra credits to stay in compliance with the team.

For the first time in a long time, I finally had something to be excited about other than a guy. I poured myself into track and it paid off. It also helped me and my mom's relationship because she was so proud of me. She was at every meet, cheering in the stands. It was like she had been waiting for me to get my life together. She had been waiting to brag about me.

That year, there was another important relationship I made in that same homeroom, and that was with the father of my child. One morning, I was sitting at my desk reading my Bible, because that was the only thing my mom let me read, and he sat near me. "Are you saved?" I asked, and he gave me a funny look. "I don't know," he replied, shrugging, and we became friends.

I made more friends with the other track girls that year, and my mom started letting me go back out. My self-esteem was being restored. I became a straight-A student all over again. I was still wearing my braids, but I wasn't hiding beneath them. They were optional and convenient when it came to working out. I no longer felt like I needed to hide or shrink myself. Sometimes, I would wear my braids, and sometimes, I would wrap my hair, and sometimes, I would wear a ponytail. I kept it versatile depending on my mood.

By eleventh grade, I was thriving. I ended up placing second in hurdles and third in pole vaulting at the Lake Erie League (LEL) tournament, a conference that includes high schools in the region. Maple's track team was on fire and, in addition to my personal wins, the team placed in the 4x2 and the 4x1 in the

LEL. We were champions, and because of all these wins, my popularity, once again, soared. Folks started talking to me who didn't used to talk to me and acknowledged me in the hallways when previously I had felt like a ghost. Boys who were known for only dating the popular pretty girls suddenly were approaching me. I was shocked that they were even interested but even with these new occurrences, when my social status climbed, I wasn't as aware. I watched the popular girls and felt out of place. I never felt like I fit in with them or that I was like them. I would often look around and feel like there was no one like me and that I hadn't found my tribe. Even though I had grown in self-confidence through track, I still underestimated how others viewed me. I was still wounded from the rejection of my childhood. I had always been called a white girl because of my vernacular and was consistently critiqued about how I carried myself. Some of this critique even came from family members. Some of this rejection was from the very ones who were now my fans at school. It was hard to let all that past trauma go. So much so that when I was asked to be on homecoming court my senior year, I turned it down. *Who would vote for me?* I thought. Sadly, I didn't run even though I had a good chance at winning. The other popular girls who could have won weren't able to because they didn't have the 2.75 GPA required. You also needed an elective, and I had track *and* student government. But even with turning down that opportunity, I maintained my popularity. I had always been a great dresser. One day at school, I was rocking black shorts, red suspenders, and red pumps with white and red jewelry. As I headed down the stairs some random girl said, "Ariel, your legs are fire!" I beamed. I had come a long way from that little girl who was teased for having big legs at Field Day in fifth grade. As a kid, my legs were looked at as a negative, but in high school, they became my assets. God had given me strong, large legs for a reason, and that reason was finally being revealed. I was a runner. I was so good, I was heading to compete in the Ohio regional conference where I placed that year.

It was in the midst of all of my success that D got released from jail and called. He wanted to see me. "I have track practice," I said, not flinching. This was major. Before he was locked up, I couldn't say no to that man, but now, I was in a whole different head space. I had a new bestie named Chante, and we were kicking it hard. We were going to teen clubs, and I was meeting new guys every weekend. I was finally comfortable with myself and stopped being so obsessed with critiquing my appearance. Boys were constantly affirming my body whenever we went out, and I knew I had options. D was no longer my only option. It was like he wanted us to pick up where we had left off, but thank God, I had transformed in the eight months he had been gone. I'm sure it was my mother's prayers. I was in such a dark place when I dated him, and nothing seemed to be getting me out of it until I started running. I became obsessed with track. My personality always has to have a goal and something to be obsessed with. Unfortunately, before track, and even when I got older, my obsession was with men and pouring into *them*. But with track, I started pouring into *me*.

Maybe because I was in a better head space with my self-esteem, self-value, and appearance, I was able to better juggle my next relationship and not completely lose myself. Unbeknownst to me, that boy that I met my tenth-grade year who I became friends with while reading my Bible had been liking me for years. While I was excelling academically and in sports, he had been monitoring me. It wasn't until our twelfth-grade year that he had his friend approach me. I had just finished track practice and was still on the field when this guy said, "My boy Chris likes you." Confused, I looked at him. "Who's that?" He said, "Don't try to play me! You know Chris," but I had no idea who he was talking about. Other than tenth-grade homeroom, I had barely seen

Chris all of eleventh grade. That next day, I saw him at lunch and realized he was the one his friend was talking about. I walked up to him and said boldly, "Do you like me?" Though he was caught off guard, he replied quickly, "Yes." "Why?" I asked, genuinely confused. Chris was quiet and shy. He played basketball but kept to himself other than that. I was more outgoing and social and felt like we were super different. He looked at me and said, "I just do." We went to sit down at lunch, and it was like being in a scene from "High School Musical". All of a sudden, the whole lunchroom was staring at us. I felt myself grow warm. I was immediately embarrassed. I do not like a lot of attention.

"They're staring," I whispered to Chris, sneaking glances around the cafeteria. "Why is that?" He shrugged. But then a girl came over to our table, trying to start something and probably thinking she was about to mess up our little impromptu date. "Are you dating Ariel now?" she asked Chris with her back to me, a blatant sign of disrespect. One thing I love to do is be a little petty when the situation calls for it. I loudly responded, "Yes!" just to see what she would do. Just as I thought, she turned and walked away.

After that, Chris and I were inseparable for 11 years. What can I say? I love love. I love consistency. Structure and routine make me feel safe, and that's probably instilled in me from the routine I had as a child. Chris and I soon fell into a routine. After school, he would have basketball practice at Stafford Park while I had track practice, and afterward, we would meet up. Our moms loved us too. His mom loved me, and my mom loved him. But Chris's home life was rough. Sadly, his mom developed a drug addiction when he was in his early teens. That made his life hard at home. His dad was always working and trying to monitor his mom while his mom was constantly stealing from them to support her habit.

Our very first date was in Chris's house, huddled beneath

blankets watching a tiny, boxed TV. The only light in the whole house was from the TV. There was no electricity due to unpaid bills, and they had an extension cord running to the abandoned house next door to steal electricity. We were shivering under that blanket in Cleveland's brutal winter. Other girls probably would have fled, but I'm a softy when it comes to a good heart. Chris was a good person, and he accepted me completely for who I was. Others always seemed to expect me to conform to their idea of who they wanted me to be. Until Chris, I never felt like I fit in and thought I needed to compromise to do so. With Chris, I never had to conform. He was super sweet, patient with me, and a very hard worker.

Throughout our high school career, Chris was constantly tired, and it took me a while to learn why. To support his family, he would work a full-time job after school at a local factory. He was a year older because he had failed a grade, so he was already 18. He worked second shift, would get off at 11 pm, then wake up for school the next day, go to basketball practice, and go back to work. It was crazy. He was a whole grown man as a teenager. To make matters worse, his own mother kept stealing the money he was working so hard for. He and I would fall asleep on the couch at his house and wake up to her rummaging through his pants pockets for money. My heart broke for him.

One day, he called and asked if my mom could give him a ride to work. "What happened to your car?" I asked. Chris had a 1980s maroon Buick he had taught me how to drive in. "My mom let the dope boys rent it out and they stripped the column," he mumbled. His own mother had stolen his car and left him incapable of taking care of himself. That's the kind of situation Chris was in. He had no one to parent him. I was the only person in his life who was any kind of support. It was for that reason that when I was offered track scholarships to Xavier University, Robert Morris University, and Notre Dame College my senior year of high school, I chose Notre Dame to stay close to home. Chris needed me. He encouraged me to leave, but there was no way I could. I was in love.

Chris and I had a good situation for a minute. I had a dorm room at college which I initially shared with a roommate, but, when my boyfriend kept sleeping over, there were some problems, even though my roommate's boyfriend was often over as well. For a while, Chris wasn't allowed over, but then my roommate fell into some academic violations which caused her to move out. This allowed Chris to stay with me permanently second semester.

We fell into a routine where Chris would work while I would go to classes and practice. I had a scholarship for the 4x1, 4x2, and hurdles and carried on my academic and athletic success into my freshman year of college. But just like before, I had issues making friends. There was some bullying in my first quarter from the other girls on the track team because they felt I was too cheerful. I came from Maple Heights where we rooted for our teammates. We had a mindset that we were winners at Maple, but these girls were rougher than my former teammates. They would cuss me out when I cheered for them. "We tired. We don't wanna hear that sh*t!" they growled. Again, I didn't fit in. Though for most of my childhood, I had lived in the hood, I was never really from it. My mom had protected me and provided for me, so my mentality was different. Because of her protection, I had been kept from a lot that would have hardened me and stolen my naturally bubbly personality. As a result, I hadn't developed a rougher persona like my teammates. But not fitting in with them didn't stop me from killing it at track. I ended up going to Nationals for hurdles. I was on fire. Plus, not having friends wasn't anything new to me. For most of that semester, Chris was my hangout buddy until he started having to pick up extra shifts to make ends meet. Suddenly, he wasn't available as much. I was sitting at lunch one day alone and one of the track girls came over. "Hey, come sit with us." That was a turnaround moment, and I finally found acceptance with them.

Life in college became a smooth ebb and flow, and my body was at its peak. At that point, I was doing two-a-days where I was working out twice a day. That meant I was burning twice the normal number of calories I would have in just one workout. My mindset around food had already become that food was fuel but now it changed even more. I started believing I could eat whatever I wanted because I was working out so much. We had an all-you-can-eat cafeteria at school, and I would load up on desserts. I had always been a dessert person and daily had my standard two pieces of cake. My mom would drop $250 in my bank account every month, so I would use it for all of my favorite foods. Track became a mental Band-Aid in regards to my nutrition, and I had yet to learn that you cannot outwork a bad diet.

It was the top of my sophomore year in the middle of October when I would have a rude awakening that would lead me to this understanding. My boyfriend and I had still been living together but at the time we were broken up due to a big argument. The breakup was more from growing pains than anything else. There was nothing major that happened. We were basically just getting on each other's nerves and having personality clashes. This particular day, I was going about my business practicing for track, but for some reason, I was exhausted. I've always been a high-energy person, so feeling drained like that was outside of my personality. Often in practice, our team would run repeat 400s, and that was nothing for me. Afterward, I would ask for more. But on this day, we had repeat 200s and I was behind everyone. I was looking around like, *Wow! What is going on? I must have the flu.*

My coach said, "Baker, are you ok?"

Am *I ok?* I was thinking, bewildered.

That evening, I went to my mom's house and mustered up

the courage to take a pregnancy test. I sat in the bathroom and read the results at least three times out loud. "Plus-minus means not pregnant. Plus-plus means pregnant." I stared at my results and looked at the instructions again, repeating them but not comprehending what I was seeing and reading. But no matter how many times I read the instructions, it did not change the result. At just 19 years old and a sophomore in college, I was pregnant.

Chapter 6
BABY MAMA

By the time I got pregnant, I had been having unprotected sex for more than a year, but for some reason, getting pregnant was never a real possibility to my 19-year-old brain. I was focused on track and school. At the time, my boyfriend and I were broken up, so I *really* wasn't expecting it. He was busy, I was busy, and though we still lived together, we were doing our own thing. I never fathomed that this would happen with someone I was no longer dating.

When I came out of that bathroom in shock, gripping the positive pregnancy test, my mom stood in the living room looking at me. "What's wrong?" she asked. I muttered the words I never thought I would at 19 years old. "I'm pregnant." But, to my surprise, she didn't flinch. "I know. Ariel, look at your stomach." She pointed to the small bulge in my mid-section pressing against my tight-fitted sweater dress. "You been having that bump for a while."

It was clear as day that I had *something* going on down there. But—*why didn't anybody tell* meee*???!* I wailed in my mind. Thankfully, my mother was supportive, and that was one less battle I had to fight. The bigger battle was telling Chris. I was so scared to make that phone call and have him come over. Maybe, for that reason, his response caused burning, hot anger to bubble up in my heart.

I ended up inviting Chris to my mom's house, and we sat down in the living room. My face was hot, I was so nervous! "I'm pregnant," I finally said. All the butterflies in my stomach swarmed at full speed. Chris looked unsurprised, but his first words shocked me. "Yeah, I figured. When are you going to get an abortion?"

I couldn't believe that was his response. How could he so quickly jump to that conclusion? It wasn't like we were a one-night-stand situation. We had been in love and were in a committed relationship for over a year, for God's sake. How could he be so quick to throw the possibility of our conceived child away like that? These were the thoughts running through my mind. But what really solidified my choice was him insinuating that I didn't have one. Yes, I wanted to keep all my options open, and that meant I didn't want abortion to be my only one. I dug in my heels and looked at him, stone-faced. "I'm *not*," I said, chin jutted out. At that moment, my mind had been made up. Just because he said I shouldn't have my child, I knew that I should. "But," Chris stuttered, "Why would we have it when we're not together?" I didn't care what Chris said. The fact that some man was going to take away my choice was more reason for me to use it.

Unfortunately, my decision to keep my child was a lonely one. There were many in my ear telling me I needed to get an abortion. Folks kept saying I was the track star in high school and they expected better from me. "We counting on you to do better, Ari. We don't want you to lose your status and success," they said as they shook their heads in disappointment. I was so ashamed.

Chapter 6

Even my own internal narrative haunted me. *I'm not a baby mama. And for damn sure not to a man who's gonna leave me!*

Everyone was telling me to get an abortion. I knew that it was a huge sacrifice to keep my child. I was a prospect to be in the Olympics and had people scouting me. I was slated to win Nationals. My future was promising but I stuck to my conviction. In some ways, I made the choice to keep my child out of spite due to the naysayers, and I'm not even a little ashamed to admit it. I chose my child over the future I could have had in track, but I don't regret it one bit. Choosing my child's life was one of the best decisions I ever made.

There was at least some relief with my track coach who said that whatever I decided, he would support. Because I chose to keep my baby, I was only able to practice track up to my fourth month. I was a hurdler, so training longer than that was out of the question. For a while, I was doing what I could on the team while trying to wrap my brain around being somebody's baby mama. Being a baby mama was never what I had envisioned. Chris and I were going through the normal breakup stuff where he was talking crazy to other females, and I was snooping through his social media finding messages then confronting him about it. I was so scared to have this child alone. But by the time I was benched for track and was well into my fourth month of pregnancy, I had moved into my mom's house. Thankfully, Chris had snapped out of it. He went from not reaching out to calling and checking up on me, wanting to know about the pregnancy and my well-being. By the time I started showing, he started spending the night again. Since he turned his attitude around and we got back together, he moved in with my mom too. We were all preparing for the baby with our new living situation.

Even though I couldn't run, the school let me keep my track scholarship. Still, it wasn't long before I fell behind in classes. I was always so tired, and I just couldn't seem to keep up. I was, however, obsessed with working out. I think I feared I was going to gain a whole bunch of weight and not be able to lose it, so the energy I did have went into going to Bally Total Fitness. The problem was I reverted back to my old eating habits. I was so used to having track practice to fill up my time and then my track friends to hang with, but once I moved off campus and was benched, all that stopped. It wasn't long before I became lonely and bored. All of my friends were practicing or partying or going to class, and I wasn't on campus anymore, so I wasn't a part of any of that. I went from being busy from going to class, doing schoolwork, and training up to four hours a day to being a stay-at-home girlfriend, sleeping all day and waiting for Chris to come home. Once he did, we would go to Bally's to workout, which was a flailing attempt to recapture some sense of normalcy that track gave me. But after our workouts, we would head right across the street to B&M's Barbeque. Like clockwork, I would scarf down a Polish Boy and two corn beef sandwiches. Then, that *same* night, I would tell Chris, "I'm hungry again." We would head right back out for a pepperoni pizza at Donato's right next to B&M's. That was our ritual at least 3-4 times a week. It wasn't long before the pounds started piling on. I was 145 pounds when I got pregnant, an easy size 4/5 in juniors. By the end of my pregnancy, I was 216 pounds. It wasn't until my seventh month that I blew up though. I was working on my legs on the machine at Bally's when a guy who had seen me running around the track there for the last several months came over. "Hey, are you pregnant?" he asked, staring at my belly. "Yeah," I said. "I'm in my seventh month." His jaw fell. "I just saw you last month. You doubled in size!" He was right. I *had* doubled in size. I was so big, my feet had swollen. But none of that deterred me. I just kept eating.

A typical meal in one sitting would consist of a Polish Boy, two corn beef sandwiches, and a side of fries. One time, I had

Chris look at his bank statement and we saw that he had spent his whole paycheck on me eating. It was crazy. I was out of control with my eating habits. It's common to have pregnancy cravings, but it's only recommended for pregnant women to take in about 300 additional calories daily per trimester (Medlineplus.gov). That's the equivalency of a granola bar! I was consuming an additional 2000 calories daily. Being pregnant and inactive had reignited my go-to behavior to turn to food when I was lonely and bored.

Before getting pregnant my mentality was that working out could hide my lack of discipline in eating. I had to learn the hard way that having healthy eating habits is foundational to being healthy. Track had been a major source of community and had given me structure, but while it taught me excellence in athleticism, and gave me a temporary goal to view food as fuel, once that goal was removed, (such as competing in track meets), I didn't have anything to rein in my appetite.

Just like when I was a kid, I was still hooked on my TV shows. My go-to soap operas were my companions during the day when Chris was at work and I wasn't sleeping. My only friends were Chris and those soap operas. My pregnancy was draining me so much that I barely went to class. It was ninth grade all over again where my teachers rarely saw me but passed me anyway. My pregnancy created such a drastic turn in my academic performance compared to my first semester when I had As in Organic Chemistry and other AP classes. Second semester, I popped in the day of the final, recited the answers my friend gave me beforehand, and was given a B in Organic Chemistry. That was the grace on my life. It is a miracle I'm a nurse. My teachers could have said, "We haven't seen you," but they had mercy on me and all gave me Bs because of my prior great performance and my current pregnancy status. They wanted to see me win.

On August 5, 2009, I had an emergency C-section due to

carrying my child too long. I was due in mid-July and was induced in late July. That induction was unsuccessful and was followed by a second induction which was also unsuccessful. The staff had to break my water because my baby's heart rate was accelerating and he was slowly dying. He had been in my womb so long he had a bowel movement that gave me an infection. That infection caused my vagina to swell closed after I was briefly dilated which prevented the induction from working. But I didn't know any of this. No one tells you anything when you don't know what to ask. I hadn't completed nursing school yet, so I wasn't able to be my own advocate. I was 19 years old, sitting there in pain, back hurting, scared, and my child was slowly dying. Finally, they rushed me into emergency surgery, and I gave birth to a baby boy weighing 6 pounds and 12 ounces.

Being a mother is a huge shift emotionally, physically, and mentally, and I wasn't ready for it. *Who was I?* I no longer ran track. I couldn't fit my clothes. I was a new mother and had never even changed diapers before. I wasn't getting any sleep and was constantly trying to figure out how to get my son to stop crying. Today, what I was going through is called postpartum, but back then, we didn't know what was going on with me. After rocking my son for hours, I would burst into tears. Chris would come home, take him for five minutes, and my son would fall asleep.

Is it me? I couldn't help wondering. *Am I the problem?*

I also wasn't ready for the inability to lose the weight I had gained during my pregnancy. After giving birth, I lost exactly the weight of my son: 6 pounds, 12 ounces. No extra weight came off. I couldn't believe it. I had fully expected to be a snapback, thinking that by the time school started, I would be able to run track again.

To my surprise, for months, I had so many designer clothes just sitting in my closet collecting dust. I couldn't fit any of my jeans. I had brands like BCBG and Steve Madden pumps and everything was too small. Even my shoes! I had always been into fashion and not being able to rock my clothes was a shot to my self-esteem. Though I was motivated mentally to workout so I could wear my clothes again, the exhaustion from having a C-section was brutal. Since a C-section is surgery, your body takes even longer to recover in comparison to a vaginal birth. You can't do any heavy lifting or too much walking for a long time. The other thing I was dealing with was the effects of being inactive for so long. No one told me I wouldn't be able to just jump back into working out once I was finally released from the doctor. Chris and I bought the P90X home workout, and I couldn't even do the jumps. Here I was a former hurdler, and I couldn't do a simple jump! The frog jumps, superman, and banana moves would take me out. It wasn't just the intensity, it was the endurance. I had lost all of it.

I had an experience a couple of months after giving birth that was also significant. Chris and I had done the P90X workout, and I felt so defeated by not having stamina. I was frustrated with my body for not being what I wanted it to be. After that workout, I ate and then went into the bathroom and made myself vomit. I honestly felt stupid and decided to never do it again, but I continued to struggle in my appearance.

Another part of my struggle was my mindset. I thought I could just pick up where I left off. I thought I could run a 200-meter dash eight weeks after being cleared from surgery. *Man, I'm really out of shape!* I thought, discouraged. This new body was a far cry from my old one. Before, I had abs, killed it at national competitions, and was an award-winning athlete. Now, I had stretch marks and couldn't even do a simple home workout. I soon fell into complacency.

Still, no matter how depressed I felt, I couldn't afford to bury myself in my feelings. I had a baby depending on me and I needed a plan. I finished out my semester at Notre Dame College and, just two weeks after giving birth, transferred to Ursuline College for nursing school. Right before I came up pregnant, my close friend informed me she was majoring in nursing, and I agreed to do the same. I had been a Communications major but wasn't tied to the idea. Once I found out I was pregnant, I knew I needed something secure and dependable. Nursing seemed to be my best bet.

I soon developed a routine of going to Ursuline while my mom watched my son, and Chris paid her for childcare. Having a kid reignited my drive, and I put myself on a clock. *I have two years to become a nurse*, I would think, homing in on my new goal. But unlike with track, this new goal did nothing to help me lose weight. Instead of working out and eating right, I was just trying to keep my head above water by excelling academically and being a stay-at-home mom.

Even though I was at least able to be social at school and meet other people, Ursuline was predominantly white, and I couldn't relate to a lot of my peers. My skin complexion wasn't the only thing that stood out. Those girls were rail thin. Their size zero made my size 10 look plus-sized. I became cool with one girl who was tiny and decided to go shopping with her my second semester. Bad idea. I already always felt like the fat Black girl around the girls from school, and now I couldn't fit into anything in the stores we went into! I was so broken-hearted. Shopping was always a great outlet for me, and even that had been taken away. I ended up getting an oversized shirt that day and made it into a dress using a belt. That night, I went to a male strip club with friends where my self-esteem, once again, plummeted. Guy after guy walked past me, detouring straight to my friends to holler at them. For years, I was the one with the great body. I was the girl guys wanted to talk to. That night, it was as if I were invisible.

Chapter 6

Halloween came around, and I was still carrying my extra weight. I was still cool with D's sister, and we went to a Halloween party together. I went as a sexy clown. Or so I thought. You know how sometimes; you don't really see yourself until you see yourself in a photo? We took a picture at that party, and my jaw hit the floor when I saw it. I looked horrible. My nose was still spread, my face was swollen, my belly was hanging out. I couldn't believe this was the new me. A guy-friend spotted me at the party and approached me. "Ariel, baby, you gained weight," he said. "I know!" I cried. I simply couldn't cope with this new version of myself. I didn't have any grace for the fact that some of the weight I put on was due to a pregnancy, which is actually healthy and normal. I was overly hard on myself and became obsessed with talking about the weight gain but not doing anything about it. My son's father was so patient and sweet with me. He always affirmed me and complimented me. But similar to when I was younger and my mom would try to affirm me, the words bounced right off. If a person can't see their beauty for themselves, no one else will be able to make them see it. It was like before when I leveled up with track. I was going to have to find a way to see it for myself, but it would take years for me to get there. My primary focus at this point in my life was taking care of my son.

My son was about eight months old when Chris and I got a small apartment in Parma, a suburb on the west side of Cleveland, and moved out of my mom's house. We were paying $435/month for a two-bedroom. Those were good times. Chris was the main source of income, and I was focused on finishing school and taking care of our son. We were good for a while. Chris supported me through school, and I was the loyal girlfriend. I learned to cook and would have meals ready when he got home. We had a cute little family unit going as young adults. I wasn't even 21 yet, but we had stepped up to our responsibilities.

My health still wasn't a priority though. I was surviving off typical meals Black people cook like fried chicken, spaghetti, lasagna, hot dogs, etc… Meals that make you feel full but aren't necessarily full of nutrition. I wasn't gaining weight, but I also wasn't losing, and I definitely wasn't working out. My focus was trying to maintain my 3.95 GPA. I never wanted to be the stupid Black girl since I was one of the few in my class. We were going about life that way with me being in school and Chris working when another hurdle surfaced. During this time, I had my son in childcare while I went to class and studied, and his caregiver pulled me to the side when I went to pick him up. My son has always been exceptional. He was walking at seven months old. He had even learned how to climb on top of the dresser to put his DVDs into the TV. So, when she shared that he wasn't talking to the daycare providers and wasn't saying his ABCs and numbers, I was confused. He had passed all of his milestones with his pediatrician. He definitely knew his ABCs and numbers. "He won't do them for us," she said. I called my son over. "He'll do them," I said and had him recite them for her, which he did. The next day, another woman came up to me when I was picking him up from daycare and gave me her card. "Hi. I'm here for another child, but I would like us to have a conversation." "About what?" I asked. "I think your son has some delays," she replied.

Delays? What is she talking about?

I looked over at the child the woman had been there for, and he held typical characteristics of autistic children such as a flat affect face, a glazed stare, an emotionless expression, hand flapping, etc.. "You think my son has autism?" I asked, in surprise. She nodded. "I think he might. Can we schedule a meeting?" I, of course, agreed, but when I got home after getting my son situated, I collapsed onto the ground. "God, whatever it is, give it to me instead or fix it!" I begged. I was so afraid for my son to be different. I knew firsthand this world is not nice to different people. My sister was teased and ostracized for being different. So was my grandmother. I had been raised in a home full of different people. Life was never easy for them.

At that point, I knew my son was sensitive to loud noises. I couldn't even flush the toilet without him covering his ears. The reason he learned to walk early was because he hated the texture of the carpet beneath his legs when he crawled, so he began crab walking to avoid crawling. This turned into actual walking. But even with these quirks, I only saw perfection. I shared the news from the lady at childcare with my mom, and she said, "Nothing's wrong with him." I shared it with my boyfriend, and he said, "Nothing's wrong with him." I told my stepdad, and he said, "Nothing's wrong with him." But when I looked at my son lining up his Hot Wheels on the floor and one fell out of place and *he* fell into a full-blown tantrum over it, I knew: *something is wrong with my son.*

Chapter 7
MIRACLE BABY

By the time my son was diagnosed with autism, we had moved from our two-bedroom in Parma to Bedford, a suburban city on the east side. We were only there for a month when the childcare workers first noticed something and approached me. That's when my life became a whirlwind as I fought to get him the care he needed. He had been a snowflake up until he was two years old and didn't fit the typical description the medical field had at that time of autistic children.

"Does your child give you eye contact?" specialists would ask. My son did while most children with autism do not. "Does he lack emotion?" they asked, but my son was very expressive. He was always smiling, laughing, and playing. He even had a little play buddy in daycare.

At first, I thought it was just the change in scenery that caused his shift in behavior since we had moved to Bedford. He had always been loving and joyful at home. I had no idea that at daycare he was isolating himself in a corner, playing alone. I had no idea how he presented in public. Then, at home, he suddenly stopped liking foods he had always loved because certain food smells were too much for him. His sensory needs had changed. Turning on the faucet and running water became a problem. The TV being too loud was a problem. Doctors would say, "Oh, some kids have more sensitive ears," but he would be screaming at the top of his lungs. That was more than just sensitive ears. Also, at two years old, he wasn't verbal like the other kids and was still pointing or grunting and making sounds to communicate. Others would tell me, "Oh, you know, some kids are just late developers." I didn't have other kids to compare him to but I knew something was up. Suddenly, he was checking boxes off the autism checklist.

It was my junior year of nursing school when I went to his pediatrician. She didn't give me any pushback, though she could have. He had already had some preliminary testing, and autism had been ruled out, but she was a kind woman who understood a mother's intuition. After I shared my concerns, she looked me in the eye. "If you believe he has it, I'll test him."

Once he was diagnosed, I was able to get him resources such as a behavior specialist, a therapist, funding for daycare, books and supplies, and social security income. Once I got the ball rolling, my family jumped on board, but that was a long, hard year. I was working with maternal babies at work and seeing "typical" children all the time. It hurt that my son wouldn't have that experience. Then I was on the pediatric rotation surrounded by more "typical" babies. After work shifts, I was going home, pouring all of my energy into my son who was *not* "typical." I wanted him so desperately to have a happy childhood. I never wanted him to feel out of place or like he wasn't normal. I knew he would already have it hard from the world, so I started overcompensating. I started taking him on dates and spending money on experiences like Disney on Ice. *Everything* became about my son. I spent all my time trying to teach him to read using books like "Hooked on Phonics" and "My Baby Can Read" to assist with his verbal skills. I did all of this not to make him advanced but to catch him up to his peers.

I was able to keep up my grades, but the need to focus on my son eventually wore out my relationship with Chris. We had both stopped nurturing the relationship. It simply was no longer about us. Instead, it became all about *How can we help our son?* Chris was also dropping the ball financially, and we faced a lot of financial stressors. The money issues coupled with our son's needs were taking a toll on us as a couple. I was always exhausted. There was always a decision to make regarding my son's health. Should he be on meds? If so, which ones? What pre-school should he attend? Does his pre-school have other kids with autism so he doesn't stand out? It's illegal for pre-schools to deny admittance; however, some will come up with excuses if they don't want to admit a special needs child.

Emotionally, I was tapped out. It's hard to explain how lonely you feel when your child is diagnosed. Even though I had a partner, we were processing it differently. Most dads will grieve the diagnosis with a son in a different way than a mom because they have this expectation of what having a son will be like. More than likely, a son with autism isn't going to be the star quarterback of the high school football team.

The reality was Chris and I were growing apart. My days were filled with studying, then picking our son up from daycare, and working with him to develop his verbal skills. I picked up a nursing assistant job to help with our financial struggles which meant I was going to school four times a week and working three times a week. The outside support rotated between daycare, my mom, Chris's aunt, and his mom. One of the silver linings during this difficult season was a conversation I had with Chris's mom after I gave birth. I said, "If you ever want to be around my son, you can't be on drugs." She quit crack cocaine cold turkey immediately and has been clean ever since. My mom also quit smoking cigarettes the same day I told her I was pregnant. My son's birth was a miracle in more ways than one. His birth inspired miracles, especially when it came to breaking addictions.

After the autism diagnosis, my relationship with Chris was already hanging by a thread, but then, during my senior year, things got worse. We got evicted from our apartment and had to move in with my mom. I started working weekends to catch up on our bills, but the cycle of debt continued. We were living off of check-in-advance places where the interest rates are sky high. Chris was hitting the casino more and more in response to our son's autism diagnosis and it was digging us into a financial rut. We were relying on whatever refunds I got from my Pell Grants for school. During the summer, I didn't get any grants, so we were struggling even more. For my son's fourth birthday, I was so discouraged. I only had five bucks to my name. I spent that five bucks and got him five $1 Hot Wheel cars from the dollar store. I was able to use our food stamps to get him a birthday cake and pizza from Walmart. I swore to myself I would never be that broke again. I wanted to give my son the world.

Before graduation, my student loans ran out and the school threatened to withhold my degree if I didn't pay my bill. I shoved over all the cash I had in order to graduate. Unfortunately, that meant my car got repossessed because I couldn't afford to pay the note *and* for college.

During this trying season, I became close with a friend's brother. We already knew each other, and he was someone I trusted. We connected online, and our initial connection was innocent. I will always turn to God when I'm going through a hard time, and he and I started having discussions about the Bible. Our communication and connection grew to us hanging out in person. I would be open about it with Chris because at first, I had nothing to hide. While my connection was growing with my friend's brother, my connection with Chris was null and void. Chris and I had been together for eight years but dealing with his mismanagement of funds had affected us both emotionally. He shut down after I kept trying to come up with ways to help us get financially healthier. I grew frustrated at what I perceived to be him not communicating. Every year we would alternate filing our taxes and who would claim our son. He claimed our son that year and the money was offset by the IRS. All this resulted in a brief breakup which ended in me moving out. I was done at that point and definitely wasn't looking to get involved with anyone. Still, I ended up falling in love with my friend's brother. We seemed to be on the same page and, similar to how most emotional or physical affairs happen, he offered what I was missing: someone who wanted the same things. I think we both got caught off guard with the relationship since he had recently broken up with someone else too. But when you spend that amount of time with someone, you're bound to catch feelings. This man had an impact on my spirituality since, as I stated before, our relationship started off by discussing the Bible. But there was a reason for that. Turns out he was a Hebrew Israelite. Hebrew Israelites are pretty strict with their diet, and it wasn't long before his lifestyle influenced mine. I let go of pork. I let go of shellfish. I started watching what I ate. Those changes helped me shed some of the pregnancy weight I was still holding onto. I also became more serious about my faith and at age 25 identified as being a Hebrew Israelite. While I had always prayed and talked to God, I started reading the Bible more and using it to hold myself accountable. I stopped celebrating holidays. I started implementing scriptural teachings into my lifestyle. Eating was a part of that.

Even though it wasn't the most moral decision to be in that relationship since it eventually overlapped when I started dating Chris again, it was my way of grasping for the only bright light in a brutally dark time. Outside of school, everything else felt like a battlefield. Losing weight made me feel better about myself, and that was a byproduct of that relationship. Even still, in my heart of hearts, I knew I couldn't leave Chris. I wanted my son to have a two-parent household, something I lacked for years and knew firsthand the effects of. My son already had it hard enough with his autism diagnosis and needed all of the stability he could get. But the biggest reason I knew I had to let the affair go was that even though I was in love with that man, I loved Chris even more. After all we had been through, I couldn't just walk away. I told myself we were just in a rough patch and that Chris would get it together on the financial front. I got back with Chris even though I was still seeing the other man. I could tell Chris was squinting his eyes a bit when I would tell him I was meeting my "friend." By the end of my senior year, I ended the affair and focused on graduation.

My son was five years old when I became a nurse, and our lives shifted again. I got hired at a hospital in Cleveland. I was making good enough money to contribute substantially to the household, even making more than Chris. He and I moved, this time splitting the $1,000 rent 50/50. I bought a new car. My spheres of influence were changing. My peers were middle-to-upper-class types going on vacations and cruises. I started wanting those things too. I started wanting to enjoy life with our extra cash flow. But Chris wasn't on it. He didn't want to get his passport, claiming he didn't have the funds. He didn't even want me to help him pay for it. He didn't want to relocate, and I had been wanting to move out of my city forever. Years later, he said that I changed, and he was probably right, but in my mind, I changed for the better. I wanted bigger and better. In hindsight, I can see we were just growing apart. We wanted different things out of life. It wasn't anyone's fault; it was just a natural progression that sometimes happens when two people start off together very young. There's bound to be growth and change down the line when you're starting off that young.

Chris and I became more like roommates. We were carrying out our obligations to our son, but we weren't talking about the elephant in the room. And when we did talk, we were no longer listening to each other. I started taking the trips he didn't want to go on with other friends. I had my nurse girls, and we went to Mexico and the Bahamas. I was having a blast. I had a growth mindset, and I was looking for ways to grow, whether that was in my lifestyle, in education, in motherhood by enhancing my son's development, or, especially, in my physical appearance. With my body, I had hit a plateau. Though I had seen some positive results from changing my diet to model a Hebrew Israelite's, I was still far from where I wanted to be with my weight. Around that time, my step-sister popped up 100 pounds lighter than the last time I saw her. "Girl, what happened to you?!" I said, shocked. My sister had been morbidly obese, weighing at least 300 pounds, but when I saw her, it was night and day. "I started going to this gym!" she explained. "Girl, take me with you!" I demanded, and she did. I used my very first nursing paycheck and coughed up the $30 monthly membership, then went to my first cardio class.

I was 188 pounds. Even though I was heavy, I've always been more athletic, so during the class, I was able to get my knees up higher than everyone else with the high knees. I was also able to jump higher, and I caught the attention of the two brothers who owned the facility. I had no idea they were brothers. I wasn't really paying too much attention when they surrounded me, shouting encouragement. I was just high off the adrenaline. I could feel the haters in the class though as the trainers circled me with their callouts. Other women were eyeing me. "Who she think she is?" their stares were screaming. But I didn't care. I loved it. I started living at that gym. I was 25 years old and working three 12-hour shifts throughout the week. It was nothing for me to sleep a few hours, go to the gym to workout at noon before work, and hit classes on my days off. Chris would keep our son at night, and he was at daycare during the day. I soon became addicted to working out and started going to all the classes. Then I evolved to doing two or three classes a day. In three months, I lost 16 pounds. But it wasn't enough. I needed more. I told my sister, and she said, "You should get a trainer." That was the golden ticket. She recommended one of the brothers who owned the gym, and I went to his office in the basement. "You've been at my class?" he asked, recognizing me, and I nodded. "Come to class tonight and we'll see how you do." He was vetting me. I didn't know it then, but he didn't train just anyone. If I could hang in class, that would mean I could hang with his training style. That evening, he caught me after class and said, "I'll see you tomorrow." When I started training with him, that's when I got the results I had been looking for. I was on such a roll that within three months of training, I decided I wanted to become a certified trainer. My trainer was all for it, and I became his protégé for all his trainers and clients. Whenever he was training me, he was posting me on social media, making me the example of his work. I reveled in the affirmation and applause. His approval became my number one goal, and I would jump through hoops to earn it. I didn't know this then, but my daddy issues were in full effect. I wanted so badly to have a man be dependable, reliable, and long-term. I wanted badly to have a father figure's acceptance and approval.

There were team challenges I became involved in that were similar to the teams on Biggest Loser which served as mini goals for me. We would compete to see who could lose the most weight in those challenges as a team. That's when things started getting real. I was soon engulfed in a world where people were losing weight at any cost. People were obsessed with losing weight for these challenges and I fell into the same trap. I would be in the bathroom where women were popping diuretics, laxatives, and diet pills. People were wrapping themselves in saran wrap and slapping on weight-loss creams to lose weight. We were all doing three hour-long cardio classes back-to-back.

Within months of working out consistently, I found myself at the drug store looking for diet pills that could hasten my weight loss journey. Unfortunately, while taking the pills, I didn't drink enough water, and my liver enzymes were out of whack. Your enzymes are supposed to be between 16-40 something and mine were in the 200s! I was close to liver failure and didn't realize it. My liver was almost indicative of a fatty liver. The doctors were alarmed and said my cholesterol was too high. At first, I was confused because I was working out so much, but then I realized it was the diet pills. That was when I knew I had to give them up.

That's ok, there are other ways, I thought.

Every Friday was weigh-in day, so I wouldn't eat all day Thursday, then pop a diuretic or laxative that day just so I could make sure I was either losing weight or maintaining my weight loss at weigh-in. At that point, I was working out five days a week and training clients on top of being a nurse. I would pick up my son from childcare, take him to his after-school activities, then we'd head to the gym. I'd drop him off at the gym's daycare while I trained my clients and took cardio classes. By the end of that first year, I was 142 pounds with only 17% body fat. I became *obsessed* with being thin. It's sad because I didn't see that I already *was* thin. My body dysmorphia was in overdrive and even though my stomach was flat as a board, I was too afraid to show it off. I chose instead to hide my stretch marks with sweat belts when working out. I had hit my physical peak, maybe even surpassed it, but my mindset hadn't changed. Inside, there was something still screaming that I was the ugly fat girl. Maybe that's why I freaked out one day after overeating and hurried to the bathroom to vomit. Years before, when I had tried this after having my son, for some reason, it didn't stick. But maybe because I was in this hyper-competitive atmosphere that was obsessed with being thin, this time, it did. It wouldn't be long before vomiting my meals would be my go-to method of shedding weight. It wouldn't be long before I would become a full-blown bulimic.

Chapter 8
PORCELAIN WHITE

I always had my arms hugging the toilet to be as quiet as possible in our apartment to bury the sound of vomiting. I made sure to keep the water running to help suffocate the noise. A bottle of bleach stayed ready at my side so I could erase the evidence as soon as I was done.

The first time I felt the actual addiction, it was unexpected. Since I'd purged before and never gotten hooked, I underestimated the grip bulimia could have. It was one of those holidays where my mom went in and cooked all the favorite soul foods. Chicken, cornbread, greens, dressing, baked beans, but *especially* mac 'n' cheese. I could eat a whole plate of that woman's mac 'n' cheese. And then there were the desserts. Everything she made was three-layered. Three-layered pineapple upside-down cake, German chocolate cake, banana pudding, and, of course, sweet potato pie. It was plate after plate after plate. I was socially eating, so I wasn't really paying attention to how much I was consuming. One bowl quickly turned into four. I often feel like I have the appetite of a grown man because I never really feel full, but that holiday, I had gone too far.

Chapter 8

Weigh-in day was approaching, and I had been eager to lose my last few pounds to reach my goal weight. This holiday binge was the last thing I needed. I was scared to death of my trainer's disappointment as well as the consequence of gaining weight. There was a running joke at the gym that you would pay on the Stairmaster all day, or do a thousand jumping jacks, or be forced to run all day if you gained weight. So, after overindulging at my mom's, I turned to the porcelain white toilet, thinking it would be just for that one time. A month later, that one time was followed by another time. Then once a month became once a week. Then once a day. Then, ultimately, after every meal.

There was so much pressure being a physical trainer. I had accumulated about 20 clients and was building a platform in fitness. Wherever you go, when they see your transformation, people will ask how you lost weight. That's how I started landing clients. People wanted to know my knowledge base. At first, I was just taking folks with me to class to workout, but after I got certified, things took off. When you have visibility, others start watching, and people were clocking me to see if I would stay fit. The pressure was both internal and external. I was feeding off the applause of my trainer and others which is unhealthy because I kept seeking outside approval to be happy. I was quickly caught in this cycle of doing whatever was possible to stay thin, and that meant making myself sick.

It probably sounds bad, but being a nurse was a tool I used to avoid some of the pitfalls of bulimia. My obsession with being thin was so all-consuming that instead of letting my knowledge as a nurse act as a voice of reason, I used it to trick the game. For instance, to avoid suffering from electrolyte imbalance like most bulimics, I would drink Zero Gatorade after I purged. To avoid dehydration, I would down an abundance of water. I knew that nodules could form on my fingers from my teeth scraping my knuckles, so instead of using my hands, I would stick clean toothbrushes down my throat. I even formed a little kit to keep with me when I wasn't at home and needed to vomit after a meal. That's how sick this disease made my mind. Here I was, in a profession to help heal the sick, and I was using my academic training and knowledge to feed my sickness. Like any addict, I told myself, *It's not as bad as it seems*. I told myself, *I'm doing what I need and I'm taking precautions to avoid some of the consequences*. Like every good addict, I was in denial.

In nursing school, we would visit the homes of people with eating disorders and watch them sit by the toilet for an hour after eating, fighting not to throw up. I never understood that fight until I was in that fight. Like with any addiction you have moments of clarity when you know you're in it too deep. Then there are other moments when you're lying to yourself and to others. Moments when you're telling yourself that you have everything under control. There were times my bulimia was so bad that if I could go three days without purging, I was so proud of myself. During those times I hated how enthralled I was in the disease and that I had lost all control. The irony is I turned to bulimia as a source of control. My son had been diagnosed with something I couldn't control and around age six had started developing behavior issues at school. He was still at a typical school and had become obsessed with ceiling fans. He would flee the school in search of fans, and they were calling me about his behaviors frequently because the administrators didn't know how to handle an autistic child. I myself had never really had a moment to grieve not having a typical child. I was in nursing school when he was diagnosed, so I grieved on the go. There was too much I had to do and get accomplished for my son, and my focus was on finishing school.

Nursing school was rigorous and brutally competitive. The Black women I started the program with either dropped out or graduated a semester or year behind because they had to repeat classes. I was the only one who made it in the top 10 of my class and I studied eight hours a day to make it happen. At that point, Chris and I were "hi and bye" and barely roommates. I hated coming home. Every time I came home, there was something for me to cook or clean. Then there was work. For years, I had worked so hard in nursing school only to get hired at a job I couldn't stand. Though I was making good money, the work atmosphere was racist and toxic. When I first started, I had formed a group with other awkward Black girls. I was so excited I had found my tribe. But then, one by one, they were dropping like flies due to the racist environment. I ended up being the only one left on the night shift, surrounded by white nurses who gossiped about each other and micro-managed my every move. The white nurses were so good at covering for each other and having each other's backs, but if I did anything wrong, they were down my neck.

One day, there was an issue with my work, and the nurse barged into a room I had previously been in with a patient and went off on me. "I don't know what your problem is, but you better get your shit together!" she screamed. It was so loud the patient who was outside the room pulled me to the side and said, "I heard everything she said, and if you want to report this to HR, I'll back you." I went to management and reported it. Nothing ever happened.

All around me, there was no control. Not with my son. Not with my boyfriend. Not with my job. But with my body, in the beginning, I had control. That's how addictions get you. You're in control, until you're not.

I'm a perfectionist through and through with an "all or nothing" mindset, so when things aren't *exactly* as I think they should be, I have to throw it all away and start over. That's how it was with my eating habits. As soon as I ate a donut someone brought into work, I went off the rails, eating anything and everything I could get my hands on. I would go on food binges and drive from one fast food spot to another, order everything I wanted, devour it, and drive to the next spot. When I was finally done eating, I knew I had an hour window until my body digested the fats. I knew I had 30 minutes before there was a sugar influx. If I made it to the toilet within 20 minutes, it would almost be like I had never eaten at all. That was my warped thinking.

I would cry out to God, begging Him for deliverance. "God, please take away whatever spirit this is!" I was so ashamed. I knew what I was doing was wrong, but I feverishly kept covering it up as much as I could. Some of it was the claps and approval I was getting. People were always complimenting me on how thin I was. The thinner I got, the more applause I received. I was working out three and four times a day. The more I worked out, the more I focused on my body. The more I obsessed about my appearance, the more I binged and purged. I was in a vicious state of never feeling like I was enough. I also had this internal drive to always be the best, but I never had a healthy sense of what that was. That was my downfall with fitness, always seeking perfection. Oh, I don't have abs? I need abs. Oh, these stretch marks are showing? I need to wear a waist belt. Oh, I'm 20% body fat? I need to be 17%. I had such unrealistic and unhealthy ideals. I was driving myself crazy counting calories. If I overindulged yesterday, I needed to fast the next day. If there were too many croutons on my salad, I needed to throw up. If I had oatmeal for breakfast, I needed to throw up. If there were noodles in my soup, I needed to throw up. It was a psychotic game that I could never win.

It wasn't until Chris caught me coming out of the bathroom one evening at home that I finally found freedom.

"Can we talk?" Chris said. Butterflies fluttered in my stomach as I made my way to him in the living room. I was nervous he knew my secret, but there was another part of me that didn't even care.

Look, I'm doing what I need to do right now, I was thinking. *I don't want you to know, but if you do, what's going to happen?*

Chris had always been super accommodating to me, and I was using that to my advantage. Never once did I think he would have enough ammunition to stop me from my addiction. But he pulled the one thing out of his arsenal that could. Chris said, "I know what you're doing, and it's not healthy. If you don't stop, I'm taking our son." My heart froze. My whole world was upside down, and my only real anchor in life was our son.

Once again, my son was the motivation for breaking an addiction. Just like Chris's mom and my mom, that day, I stopped my addiction cold turkey. My son did that for me. My son was the inspiration for all of us to get our lives together.

The struggle was deeper than just being bulimic though. I stopped vomiting my meals, but I turned up with other unhealthy ways of losing weight. I turned up with diuretics, with obsessing over everything I was consuming, with working out several times a day. Eating disorders are not just a physical issue. They are very much a mental health issue. How you see yourself in your eyes determines your actions. How you think about yourself dictates how you treat yourself. I was always hard on myself, whether it was about school, work, or my weight.

Outside of working out, I had no healthy outlets to deal with all of the hard stuff I had going on. The cut-throat nursing program, the racist nurses at work, the rapid decline of my relationship, the autism diagnosis, and all that that entailed. My son had started to hit himself or cause self-harm when he didn't get his way or couldn't find his words. Dealing with these new conditions of his autism was exhausting. Looking back, I can see I had been going through a nervous breakdown but was too focused on trying to survive to even notice. I was a hamster on a wheel running full speed ahead, trying to control the one thing I felt I could control: me. The gym was always my go-to safe space. It often brought me joy and made me feel like I could conquer the world. But even that would be taken away.

The day came when I gained five pounds. I had gotten on birth control because even though Chris and I's relationship wasn't the best, we were still sexually intimate and going through the motions of being together. It seemed like the weight appeared overnight. I was at the gym working out and my trainer said, "Look at you! I can't post you! You gained weight!" I was so embarrassed. I felt like shit. I had let down my trainer. I had let down myself. The weight I put on was probably barely noticeable, but back then, I only saw failure.

One thing became clear: the gym was no longer my place of joy. After that day, I decided I was done with the gym and I let go of my trainer. I also let go of being a personal trainer. Those were big moves because the gym was one of my major sources of community. I wasn't just walking away from my trainer, I was walking away from a huge part of my life. But I didn't want to be somewhere that didn't bring me joy and where fitness wasn't fun anymore. I chose me. That same week, I quit my job and my relationship with Chris. I was so burned out by the hamster wheel. I simply couldn't continue being miserable in all of these spaces.

People don't typically talk about feeling lonely in their relationship, and that's where Chris and I were. Chris had always been my best friend. I honestly feel like I had a baby with my best friend, but that wasn't enough for me to stay in the relationship. I had been holding on to him for so long because I was scared to lose that familiarity. Then, something in me switched, and I decided to do it scared. All in one week, I let go of everything except my son. By then, he was seven years old. Making that transition gave me more time to fully focus on him and get him

Chapter 8

what he needed. Finding a good school for him was priority because of the issues we were having with him escaping the typical school. I transitioned him into a school for autistic children which proved to be the best decision for him. He has been thriving at that same school ever since.

For three beautiful months, I was so proud of myself. I had quit everything that didn't serve me. I picked up a PRN job where I was a nurse on call and worked as needed. I also worked in a hospice on the weekends where I loved the work environment. I got to wear business professional attire and be cute. No more shady, racist nurses coming for me. I was able to run errands in between shifts and do what I needed for my son. Chris and I were still on good terms and co-parenting. We had always been good friends and still hung out, so, though I let go of the romantic aspect of our relationship, I held onto the part that did serve me: his friendship. I was 28 years old when I moved into my own apartment and was paying $1,300/month for a three-bedroom. I stayed in Mayfield Heights near Chris so he could easily see his son. I was maintaining my weight by using a trainer online who was sending me meal plans. I had also taken myself off the birth control to avoid more weight gain. It was a bit lonely after letting go of these huge communities in my life, but, for the most part, I was reveling in standing on my own two feet. I used a lot of that time alone to do some deep self-reflection. I had come a long way, and there was much to be proud of. I had paid for all of my furniture in full for my apartment and didn't have to put anything on credit. In the evenings, I would come home and marvel at my accomplishments. *Wow, look at me!* I thought. For the first time in my life, I was in the healthiest place I had ever been in on all fronts.

But that's when the most dangerous relationship I've ever experienced emerged. That's when I started dating a man who almost killed me.

Chapter 9
RED FLAG

For two months, we were consumed with each other. Isaiah was sweet, funny, and charming. We met at the gym in passing before I quit going, often just exchanging pleasantries. But one day, I saw online that he had a goal to lose a certain amount of weight. I messaged him that I'd treat him to a coffee if he did. It was completely innocent, and I went about my day. That was before the fallout with my community, breaking up with my longtime companion, and having so many shifts in my life. Unbeknownst to me, I was in a vulnerable state. I was scrolling on social media in my new apartment when my eyes lit up. Isaiah had posted that he lost the amount of weight he was aiming for. Instantly, I remembered the coffee I'd promised, so I messaged him and we made plans to meet. It was a great meetup, and we hit it off instantly. It was like I had known him for years and since his personality was the exact opposite of my child's father he felt like a breath of fresh air. Things slowly progressed via texting into a budding friendship. We had joked about going kayaking until he ended up inviting me. I was so excited. I loved doing stuff like that and had prayed that God would send me an active man who loved to travel. When I arrived to kayak though, I was surprised to see his cousin. His cousin turned to him and whispered, "Man, I think she thought this was a date." Isaiah's brows shot up in surprise. Later, he shared he didn't think he could even pull me and that was the reason he hadn't initially tried to. But after his cousin's comment he realized I liked him and that gave him the push he needed.

Isaiah's pursuit was exhilarating. We shared the same interests, loved working out, and connected on so many levels. But truth be told, God was trying to warn me about Isaiah on our very first date. We had driven separately to meet up to eat, and afterward, were on our way to hit another spot. I was tailing him a few cars behind when I saw the police sirens. *What's going on?* I thought. The officers pulled him over and I parked behind him. One of them told me they were taking Isaiah to jail because he had a warrant out for his arrest. *What?!* Immediately, I drove to the jail and spoke with the bondsman who gave me the amount of his bail. Without a thought, I hopped into my car, sped to the ATM, and withdrew hundreds of dollars before rushing back to the jail. I had already been emotionally committed at that point given our friendship and familiarity and felt a sense of obligation to help. When the cops brought him in, Isaiah looked at me, surprised. "How long you been here?" he asked. I was flushed with adrenaline and huffed out, "For a minute."

Yes. I bailed that man out of jail on our very first date. That may seem crazy, but everything in me wanted to prove that I was a "ride or die". I was so bruised from my last failed relationship that had lasted 11 long years. I was ready to do *anything* to make sure my next one worked. How could I put that kind of time into something that didn't last? I felt like I needed to earn my keep to ensure this next one would, and I used my money to make that happen.

For our second date, we went to the gun range. Bad idea.

Isaiah said that he was great at shooting. I'm not sure if that was true because when he took a shot, the bullet ricocheted off the ceiling and fragments of it hit the guy next to us who cried out in pain. I too felt pain and looked down at my shoulder. I had been hit! But even with these obvious warning signs, I forged ahead with the relationship. My eagerness to have a successful relationship took the lead, along with how well we got along.

Those first few months had me all in. This man adored me, and I had never been adored like that before. I even met his family super early, and, despite his initial hesitancy, his pursuit went from zero to a hundred. It was only two months into the relationship when I saw a note on my car at work. As I walked closer, I realized it was a card. When I opened it, I read his endearing profession of giving me the key to his heart. My eyes bulged at the key to his apartment tucked inside. I melted.

If only I had known what love bombing was. Isaiah and I went everywhere together and became inseparable. He was the first romantic partner where our lives were completely enmeshed. I never had someone share my passion for fitness the way that he did. We were both ancient history buffs, and I soaked up all the intellect he had on these subjects. I thought he was the best thing that had ever happened to me. As far as my body was concerned, as is typical with new couples, I gained "happy weight." I was still working out, but we were always going out to eat, and the pounds started adding up. It wasn't long until I reached the 170s. The funny thing is I wasn't that concerned about it because I was so focused on him. It's sad to say, but I loved that man more than I loved myself. I breathed for his presence. When Isaiah walked into the room, I felt alive.

It was month three when things took a turn in the relationship. I had fallen asleep in Isaiah's apartment and was jarred awake by him shaking me. Sleepily, I opened my eyes to see him standing over me, waving my phone in his hand. "WTF is this!?"

Chapter 9

Isaiah screamed, eyes raging. Confused, I squinted at him. "What? What's wrong?" "This nig*ga under yo comments!" He was upset because my ex had posted emojis with heart eyes under a picture of me in ethnic garb. I couldn't believe it. Fearful and confused, I got off the bed, trying to console him, but he was so mad and continued screaming and shouting. Before my eyes, he picked up the bed mattress, threw it against the wall, and broke the frame. Pieces flew everywhere. Trembling, I moved to the living room and leaned my back against the wall. He hurried over and punched his arm straight past my face into the wall, then fell on the couch and started crying. "Why is this happening to me? Why don't you love me?" he wailed. That did me in. Everything in me wanted Isaiah to know I loved him. I went into his bedroom and started picking up the pieces to the bed frame. It took me forever, but I put the entire bed back together. When I was done, I hugged him and we went about our day.

That experience was a huge red flag to demonstrate to me that this was not a healthy individual, but I, like so many partner abuse victims, took on the responsibility of the abuser. I felt like Isaiah's act was caused by my wrongdoing, even though I had done absolutely nothing wrong. I'm also by nature a caregiver. I see someone in pain, I want to make them better. It took me going through this toxic relationship to learn that only the person who is mentally ill can get the help they need to make themselves better. I knew this even from my battle with bulimia. I had to find my own motivation to stop purging, which was my son. But I had yet to understand this concept in a romantic relationship. Unfortunately, it would take going through more traumatic experiences with Isaiah for me to learn.

Though I stayed in the relationship, I started walking on eggshells. Isaiah's jealousy grew along with his list of dos and don'ts. We worked out together, but I wasn't allowed to make eye contact with any of the male coaches and had better not even think about speaking to them. One coach gave me a side hug to greet me, and after the workout, Isaiah started screaming in the car. "You let him touch you!" But what was I supposed to do? Be mean to a man who was being kind to me? To avoid arguments, I became antisocial at the gym. My whole body language changed. When we went to workout, I put my head down and stapled my eyes to the floor. I just wanted to have a good day, which meant I had to change my naturally bubbly personality. I became antisocial Ari while he was the social butterfly. He would go to the gym and greet everyone, especially other women. The rules he made for me didn't apply to him, and he was the king of gaslighting. It was common for Isaiah to flirt with other women and compliment their bodies right in front of me, but when I addressed him about his inappropriate behavior, it was all in my head. I was being insecure. I was seeing things.

A woman from the gym who I had caught him flirting with approached me to ask if we were even still together because of the way he had pushed up on her. I never felt so low. This man was making me into a fool. He hated that I had a friendship with my child's father, yet he could flaunt his flirting in my face whenever he wanted. To make it worse, he was hypercritical about my parenting skills even though he had no children of his own at the time. My son would flap his hands if he was upset, and I was told I wasn't a good mom. A condition of my child's autism was used as a weapon to minimize me as a parent. His putdowns constantly made me feel like a horrible girlfriend and a horrible mother. He was also super jealous of my son. I had made my son breakfast while Isaiah was asleep one day. When he woke up, it was the afternoon, and he wanted to know why I hadn't made him breakfast. I explained it was because he was asleep but offered to make him lunch. "See, this is why I would never marry you, because I could never be with a woman who would take care of her son better than me," he spit out.

With Isaiah, it was like I couldn't do anything right. But there was no one else I talked to about any of it. Isaiah was my main source of companionship, and, for a long time, I wasn't ready to leave him. Talking to others would mean I had to be ready for that. For months, I stayed isolated and locked inside this prison of a relationship wrought with excessive criticism and undeserved jealousy. The love bombing I experienced early on was the extent of Isaiah's grand gestures and after that initial two-month period there were only fleeting moments of peace were overshadowed by toxicity. Finally, six months into the relationship, I had had enough and broke up with him.

Breaking up was hard because even though he made me feel like sh*t, so much of our time was spent together, especially working out. I had lost my only consistent friend. I started ducking and dodging to avoid him at the gym. It wasn't long before the depression set in and the weight started falling off. People were pulling me aside asking if I was ok. My weight had dropped into the 140s and even though that's really low for me, I couldn't eat. I was so hurt by the breakup. From losing my closest friend. From the failed dream of finally finding love. But I was pushing through it. I was moving ahead and focusing on healing and getting healthy. I had work. I had my son. I had my sanity. Day after day, I pushed through.

I even started therapy. The thing about therapy is it's not a quick fix. For a good year I attended therapy with a caring psychiatrist to help me deal with this man I loved who wasn't loving me back. I went in for depression and anxiety, but my therapist listened to me rant from one topic to another and asked, "Have you ever been tested for ADHD?" I shook my head. "Women can be harder to diagnose because they're more hyperactive and their thoughts are displaced," the doctor explained, then gave me two tests and one assessment. Afterward, I learned I have severe ADHD. I struggle with anything that makes me sit down for too long. I struggle with completing administrative tasks. It finally made sense why I always have to have a challenge and get bored with things quickly. I have to constantly find *something* new and fresh to focus on. It also explained why I feel unworthy every second of the day if I don't have something to do. To combat it, I was unknowingly managing my symptoms through extreme workouts and controlling my diet.

Therapy was one of the best decisions I ever made and helped to shift my mindset. I started off three times a week because I was determined to make healthier choices and gradually dwindled them down to twice a week and then once a week.

But while I was making steps to take care of my mental health, I knew Isaiah was not. In the course of our relationship, some of the comments he made had me concerned for his wellbeing once we broke up. While dating, I would often struggle with anxiety over him not being in a good head space if I left him. I can see now those comments attributed to me staying in the relationship. About six weeks after the breakup, I started doing wellness checks and would drive by Isaiah's house to make sure he was ok. If the light was on, I would know he was good.

One evening, I was at the mall with my sister and felt strongly I needed to check on him. I hadn't heard from him when usually I would get a text saying he missed me and updating me on difficulties he was having in life such as a job loss or financial struggles. I became worried about his mental health. He was ignoring my calls, so I decided to visit. Isaiah answered the door, looking drunk, high, and in desperate need of a haircut. Apparently, he had just been sitting in the dark when I showed up. I stayed so long, that I ended up falling asleep there and woke up to him hitting me with a pillow. "What's wrong?" I asked. "You need to go!" He commanded, eyes blazing. "Why?" But before I could even think, he picked me up and started carrying me out of the house. Isaiah lived upstairs in a two-family duplex, so we had to go down the stairs for me to leave. When we reached the top of the steps, he bear-hugged me while I struggled to grip the sides of the doorway. Then he put his forearm up to my neck and started choking me. My head fell back, and my eyes shot to the ceiling as I started blacking out. My feet were dangling in mid-air as he continued to choke me with his arm. He then tried to throw me down the stairs, but luckily, I caught myself falling forward. I fell to the floor and started crying. That's when I saw the gun in his pocket. Isaiah started crying too. We were like that for hours. Just sitting there, crying. It was pitch-black when that incident happened and by the time we got up, it was light outside. But it didn't feel like it had been hours. It felt like time stood still.

"Are you hungry?" I finally asked. He said he was, so I took him to eat. While we were eating, he said, "Trying to get you out the house, I broke my game piece," so I took him to get a new controller for his game. When I dropped Isaiah off at his house and he got out of the car, he said, "Stay up." After all of that, that's what he said to me. That's when I knew, *I love him, but he doesn't love me.*

After that, I left Isaiah alone. A few weeks passed, and one evening, he showed up at my door. "What are you doing here?" I asked, confused. He gave me some spill about how he wanted to get his life together. He was enrolling in the military. He was ready for therapy. He was ready to be the man I wanted him to be. I swallowed the whole song and dance and agreed to give us another try. I started prepping him for the military, taking him to his appointments. I even paid for his therapy. Things were good for a little while. Until they weren't. He got rejected from the military because he was overweight. I love to turn lemons into lemonade. "That's ok," I responded. "We can get healthy together!" I had been doing a hip-hop step aerobics class, and Isaiah had been fighting me on learning it. Finally, he caved, and I taught him how to step. But the chaos of his life unraveling continued despite these healthy changes. His car was always breaking down, and I was constantly paying to repair it. I would take him everywhere in mine, but an argument would inevitably surface. We would be in the car, and he would pick a fight, then throw his phone out the window. I would buy him a new one. He couldn't keep a job and kept getting fired. It wasn't long before he got evicted from his apartment. His temper was constantly on ten. After an argument one day, he threw his PlayStation on the ground and shattered it. I went out and bought him a new one. I always felt responsible.

The problem was I was fixated on those first couple of months of the relationship. I was fixated on the love bombing stage, but it was never like that again. That's the stage where abusers reel you in, and once they know they have you, all hell breaks loose. And that's what had happened. Hell was breaking loose. Once he got evicted, Isaiah was always at my apartment. Then Covid hit. Things got worse. Everyone was either off work or working from home. I was still a nurse, so I was still working my shifts. I also started hosting step parties at my house where people would come over to do hip-hop step. My house became the workout house.

One evening after a work shift, I came home thinking I would meal prep. I had bought so much food. Wings, veggies, ground turkey, but there was nothing. I stared inside the fridge confused. Everything was gone. "Babe, where's the food I had?" I asked. Isaiah was on the couch playing his video game and barely looked up. "I don't know," he grunted, shrugging. Confused, I checked the trash. Nothing. The house smelled like something had been cooking so I knew he was lying. "Did you eat everything?" I demanded. He looked up from his game. "So, what if I did?" I couldn't believe it. This man had the audacity to eat all my food that I paid for and not even say sorry. "What you gone' do about it?" he added. I was done.

I can't do this anymore.

"Leave," I demanded, but he refused and overrode all of my authority. Days prior, I had given him a house key and somehow, he had gotten it into his mind that this was his house. I called the police. They showed up but were absolutely no help. "Ma'am, we can't have you evacuate him, and he has nowhere to go, and we're in the midst of Covid. You gave him a house key, so he has access to this home. We recommend you stay on opposite sides of the home." Yes. The police department actually told me that. My life was in danger from a man whose name was not on my lease, and they actually said he had a right to be in my home because he had a house key. It was at that point I feared for my life. If the law enforcement, who were paid to protect and serve, weren't going to protect me, who would?

I can't live like this, I thought when the police left. I decided to go live on social media. Appealing to my community, I explained my situation, that I had been living with a man who had proven to be dangerous, and the police had done absolutely nothing about it. Everyone responded in support and encouraged me not to renew my lease which was up in just a few weeks. That night, I rented a U-Haul online. The very next morning at 6 am, 12 friends surprised me by showing up to move me out of my house. I was shocked. One male friend, who I had cut off due to the relationship, was right there. "We moving you out!" he declared. And they did. Folks started helping me pack. I had boxes everywhere from friends bringing them. My mom was helping too, and we went to pick up the U-Haul. She agreed I could move in with her. The whole time we packed, Isaiah taunted me, making comments and harassing me, but I ignored him. Then he started flipping over trash bags and all the boxes, making a mess. He was enraged. I had to clean up everything, but that didn't stop me. I was leaving.

After two years, I was finally free of that relationship, and it was due to the help of community. Partner abuse victims are often isolated in their situation, and during the pandemic, many were stuck in the same household as the person who was endangering them. It was my community that motivated me to leave. It was my community that gave me the out. I left my apartment two weeks shy of my lease ending and told Isaiah he could have it.

Sometimes in our lives, we can't move forward into something positive until we let go of something negative. Just one week after I made the choice to release that toxic relationship for good, I got a text message from my old personal trainer's brother.

"Hey Ari, would you want to do step in the basement for my company?"

What else am I going to do but sit around and be fat? I thought and immediately agreed.

That was the beginning of a new season of my purpose. That's when I became a big stepper.

Chapter 10
BIG STEPPER

Step saved me. After I fled to my mom's, I was depressed. I couldn't believe I was almost 30 years old and back living with her. Thankfully, she was supportive, but I was still broken up inside. How had I gotten it so wrong? How had I spent a total of 13 years with two men who were not it? And then, to go from one man I thought was not it to a man who put his hands on me. What was wrong with me? That's where my mind was when I got that text inviting me to do step. Step became my weapon for fighting depression.

For four days a week, my old trainer's brother, who was the head instructor, did the callouts while a handful of us stepped in a small basement in a house not too far from where I lived. I needed it. Everything was still shut down from Covid and no gyms were open. I had absolutely no social outlets except for step.

The group I stepped with was cool and we had a blast. *I get to workout for free and have fun? I'm not just sitting around getting fat? Say less.* It was the best of both worlds. Doing step became the thing I looked forward to. Then we ended up adding a day and stepping five days a week, sometimes twice a day for fitness challenges. I had no idea at the time the kind of online visibility the brand was getting from streaming classes, or even my own personal visibility. I was just stepping. But then, my social media started popping. Daily, I was getting 50 followers added, 100 followers added. It was crazy. Still, I never looked at the brand's social media numbers and had no idea the videos of us stepping were exploding. Millions of viewers were watching us step worldwide!

When we began the videos, it was very basic moves, but as we advanced, I started putting my own spin on things and adding moves. I'm a creative by nature, and my ADHD has to keep things fresh. My style was welcomed by the head step instructor and his team, and they moved me from the front of the videos to the back. They did this to capture my feet on the back camera which showed viewers how to do moves from their position and angle. Being moved to the back was cool with me. The less attention, the better. Being in the back gave me space to be my full creative self and do me. I was thriving.

During this time, I was sitting pretty at 148 lbs. in my thin state. My body was bodying. Not too long after stepping, I also got involved in a super competitive running club and became dedicated to winning races. On a typical day, I would train and run five miles at Euclid Creek for competitions. There were days I would walk a mile, run four, *and* do step. My body was fire. Similar to my track days, I was pretty much able to eat whatever I wanted because I was doing so much cardio. But this time, my diet was healthier because so many restaurants were closed. The pandemic was one of the most structured, disciplined seasons of my life. While others were struggling with inactivity, I was staying active. While others were shut-in, I had step. For the first time in my life, I was also happily single. I had a few dates here and

Chapter 10

there, but for three solid months, I had no interest in anything more and I wasn't pressed to be in a relationship. For the first time in a long time, I was focused on me.

Another opportunity soon emerged. The company I stepped for had been certifying new instructors every weekend. I hadn't really been paying too much attention and didn't know that certifications were booming. The head step instructor was out sick, and his manager asked me to be the stepper to demonstrate the moves for new step instructors getting certified. When the manager asked if I would step to demonstrate the moves while she did the callouts, I said, "Sure, no problem." In exchange, she offered to certify me as an instructor. "Wow. Ok. But I don't know if I really want to be an instructor," I replied honestly. I had never considered becoming an instructor and felt butterflies just thinking about being in front of everyone teaching a class. But she waived away my concerns. "Girl, you should definitely instruct! I'm gonna make you an instructor!" And that was how I became a step instructor.

Sometimes, purpose looks like that. You can be in your flow, living your life, having no idea there's something missing, and then, when you discover it, you wonder how you ever went without it. And just like what happened to me, sometimes purpose takes someone else saying, "Hey! I see something in you!" And them looking at you helps you see there's something in you too. I believe God used her in that moment to say, "Ari! Hey! Pay attention! There's something in you!"

Still, it took the manager following up with me a week later for me to make any real moves with my certification. "When are you going to teach your first class?" she pressed. "First class? You mean for the instructor thing?" I replied. I was still hesitant about putting myself out there like that. "Yea, girl," she said, and her push motivated me to move forward.

I locked in a gym and picked a date for my first class for a few weeks out. Once I posted my flyer online, I started practicing callouts. Callouts are the step moves every instructor announces to direct the attendees in what moves to do. It was one thing to be a stepper, but a whole other ball game to announce the callouts. When you're stepping, you don't have to worry about saying callouts, but when you're an instructor, you have to pace the callout at the right moment for the stepper to know which move to do on beat. For three weeks, every time I heard a song on the radio we stepped to in class, I would practice the callouts. That's how I trained myself to be an instructor.

Suddenly, it was game day. I've always had to fight feeling like people won't show up for me. Like people won't support me. But my very first day teaching as a step instructor blew all of my fears out the water. The gym was packed! Everyone showed up. Even in the midst of Covid, people came with masks on, and we had them sign waivers to avoid liability. Folks didn't care. They wanted to step! If I ever needed validation that I was called to be a step instructor, that was the day I received it. I had only stepped for six months in that tiny basement before I became a certified instructor. I hadn't searched out being an instructor but it had found me, and it had found me fast. In no time, doors of opportunity began flying open and instructors at other gyms invited me to teach step. I started teaching more advanced moves and saying the callouts faster. Within six months, I became a traveling instructor and would drive out of town to teach. The gym would ask what I was charging, and I would split sales 40/60, only requiring that my travel costs be covered. People started telling me I was their inspiration to be an instructor. I was shocked. I had barely agreed to be certified, but this was clearly a huge part of my purpose. Folks started recognizing me from being online, and I became "The Step Girl." At first, I was only teaching two days a week, but about a month in, I was teaching four. I was soaring.

Around the time I was taking off in step, I started seeing someone. He and I met at the gym. I was looking for a clip to hold the weight on my bar, and he went out of his way to find me one. His eagerness was endearing, and I also couldn't help but notice how fine he was. "I would love to take you out," he said and then knocked me off my feet when I met him that very day for a picnic spread on the beach. The man was a romantic through and through and was clearly not playing any games with me. I was impressed. But, while the conversation was great, the food was good, and the ambiance was amazing, his being extra-polished was a little off-putting. I like my men masculine, but he was well-manicured with a flawless beard. I ended up asking the question out loud that I had been thinking. "Are you gay?" He laughed and said no. I took him at his word and chalked my perception up to my own trauma.

We had a great time dating. He was stable, consistent, and loved doing all the things I loved. We traveled, worked out, and were in sync in so many ways. He had a kid, and I had a kid. We were in bed by 9 pm and up at 5 am drinking tea on the balcony, watching the sunrise. He was supportive of my dream and even purchased stepboards for my classes. He cooked for me often and was patient and kind. It was everything I needed. But coming off that toxic relationship with Isaiah opened my eyes. I couldn't give of myself to the extent I gave to Isaiah. Giving so much of myself without limit burned me. So, this time, I took my time emotionally. We didn't become official until about six months in. Now, I was dating for stability. Now, I was dating for companionship and building a successful future together. Now, I was dating smart.

This man was checking off all my boxes. He was everything I desired to manifest. We looked good together. We were fly. We were accomplished. It was the most mature, peaceful relationship I had ever been in. I was happy.

Unfortunately, my happiness with step took a nosedive. At practice one day I made a comment that was taken wrong by the manager. One of the other high energy steppers made a suggestion that we should do a class highlighting the high-energy steppers. I agreed and suggested four steppers who should be featured which did not include the manager. She said, "So you're saying I'm not high-energy?" I was surprised she took offense since she was not a stepper and I was only referring to the steppers. I responded, "No, that's not what I said." Even though I tried to clear it up, after that day, we never spoke in person again. It was disappointing because I thought we had a good relationship. After all, she was the one who had encouraged me to become an instructor. But I also felt I had never been a "girls' girl," meaning I didn't kick it with a lot of women. Growing up I was always switching best friends or didn't fit into a clique. Since I had often had issues with females, when I was ignored in step class, or felt like I wasn't allowed to even speak, I decided to just focus on the workout. I ignored the bad energy and kept it moving. My mindset was, *I came here to step*. But then, I noticed the manuals were instructing rules that only pertained to me. Like, only the master trainers were allowed to travel. There were only a few master trainers, and I was the only one who wasn't a master trainer who was traveling. Suddenly, I wasn't allowed to travel to teach my classes? Suddenly, the instructors weren't able to issue callouts that weren't in the manual which is what I had always done and was even previously affirmed to do? I started getting emails that I couldn't do x, y, and z and was constantly out of compliance. Suddenly, I couldn't do me.

I'm the type to keep it professional even when my world is crumbling. With all of these blatant attacks at bullying me, I showed up. I would turn up at step and then go home. I knew the issues were just with this one individual, so I tried not to let her sway me. Still, it was hard when I had previously felt so alive and energized in that environment. Things went on like that for several months and, once again, working out just wasn't fun anymore.

Dang. I came down here just so I wouldn't get fat during Covid, I would be thinking. Now, I'm dealing with bullying and a hostile workout environment. Now, I don't even know if it's ok for me to open my mouth and speak. I ended up decreasing my step days from five days a week to two. I also knew I needed to find a new gym to teach at due to the bullying. I went to my old trainer and told him what I needed, and we were able to make amends after the fallout between us. I've been teaching my classes at his facility ever since.

The other issue that surfaced with becoming a big stepper was the added pressure of being in the public eye. One day, I was put in front near the camera, and a comment was made on the social media live that said, "Congratulations, Ari!" The person thought I was pregnant. Even though the producer erased the comment, it stuck with me. I became too afraid to eat before a recording and was super conscious of the type of shorts I wore. I never wore shorts that were too tight on my belly or made me look pregnant. I was so thin and small back then, it was nuts. I had a cardio body, but it was never enough. It seemed like I was always apologizing for my weight.

Even with all the drama with step, I still had work to keep me busy. I became a traveling nurse, and every weekend, took the four-hour commute to Cincinnati. My son, who was 11 at the time, would stay with his dad or my mom during my shifts. Travel nursing during Covid was lucrative and enabled me to continue meeting my financial goals. I even bought my first house! A three-bedroom, two-bath in Lyndhurst. In the same week, I upgraded to a new vehicle. Even though I was blessed to be in a position to keep my job during a worldwide pandemic, it was a lot of work, and I was always exhausted. I had started talking about leaving work to be a full-time trainer but hadn't yet made any moves.

It was in 2021 around my 31st birthday that everything rumbling beneath the surface came to a head. I was still happy in my relationship, but there had been a few items that were cause for pause. My boyfriend's son had been caught in a string of crimes during the pandemic, and my boyfriend was taking it hard. I noticed that the more hiccups occurred with his son, the more anger he demonstrated. Early on, he had shared that he had a prior domestic violence situation. He explained that it was due to him bear-hugging his ex too hard until she passed out. As a result, he had weekly meetings with a probation officer. I also knew he'd spent a few months in jail, although I didn't know why. It wasn't enough for me to walk away, but it was enough for me to keep one eye open. I knew at the very least he had a hard time managing his emotions. One time when he got upset about his son, he banged his fist on the desk and punched in a wall.

I cared about this man, but the things that surfaced about him had me keep ten toes on the ground. I'd learned that much from my prior abusive relationship. I'd learned that much from doing therapy. In therapy, I developed a new mindset that influenced me to make better choices in my relationships after Isaiah. I learned that my daddy issues had resulted in a "savior complex" which caused me to keep wanting to save men who didn't want to be saved. I also realized my life seemed to always revolve around men. Whether it was my old trainer, his brother, the men in my life who I dated, or issues from my father. I wanted better for myself. I wanted to be healed, and I was on that road to healing. But do you know how sometimes, God will bring back around the same situation to test you and see if you've really learned? That's what happened with this guy.

Chapter 10

For my 31st birthday, I took a trip to Florida for a spiritual reading, and this woman read me from cover to cover. "Has the man you're dating been in jail?" she asked. I slowly nodded. "He's not gay, but he has slept with other men in prison," she revealed. My eyes widened as I thought back to my first impression of my boyfriend. On and on she went like that, sharing explicit details about him that I had either already known or suspected. It blew my mind. I had no real proof that he would or could harm me, but I couldn't deny the accuracy of what she said. "You've got to get out," she said, warning me about his abuse. What made all these details significant was that my boyfriend was a nationally qualifying MMA fighter. There were instances where he would hug me so tight it would take my breath away. These instances were triggers of the abuse from Isaiah. Prior to my spiritual reading I would minimize them, but the writing was on the wall. And then, she really got me. The reader told me that I needed to leave my job. That was something that had already been stirring in my heart. And then she said, "You know that group you're working out with? They don't support you." My heart dropped. I was already going through so much with the manager that I couldn't deny her words. I knew in my heart of hearts everything she said was true.

So, I made another big move in my life. The huge shifts I'd made three years prior were the same ones I began again. I quit my relationship, I quit my job, and I started realizing I needed to quit my workout community. These were not easy decisions to make because I liked my boyfriend *a lot*. I may have even loved him. But I had already experienced the effects of not following my instincts when I didn't leave Isaiah after God showed me the warning signs.

When I got off the plane from my trip, my boyfriend was right there waiting for me. He was so happy to see me, but I knew I had to kill his dreams. We got in the car, and I started questioning. "Tell me what happened *foreal* with your ex." He was quiet. "Have you ever been with a man?" He was quiet again. That was enough for me. "Look, this feels crazy, and I know I don't have a lot of evidence, but I got to stop messing with you." Of course, he tried to talk me out of it, but there was no going back. I was done.

Not too long after we broke up, I received more confirmation that I had made the right move. Chris was talking about my dating this guy to a coworker who just so happened to be the best friend of my boyfriend's ex. What were the odds?! When Chris showed my boyfriend's picture to the coworker, he said, "She has to stop talking to him immediately," and filled Chris in on how abusive my boyfriend had been to his best friend. The coworker also gave Chris his best friend's number for me to talk to her, which I did. I found out the supposed bear hug my boyfriend gave her was actually him strangling her. Everything was filed publicly, and police reports confirmed that he had tried to kill her multiple times and frequently beat her. He had even tried to kill himself and beat the mother of his child. It was as clear as day that I had escaped another close call with a dangerous man. Once again, God spared me.

Over a year went by after my birthday trip, and I was still doing step. I had spent a year and a half in this hostile situation and endured with grace, never once complaining. But finally, I knew I couldn't stay any longer. In the spring of 2022, I had a conversation with the head trainer and explained that the situation with the manager was still continuing. The first time we talked, there was no outcome, but this time, he had the manager call me. We had our very first conversation in over a year. Unfortunately, it didn't rectify anything. There had been a new manual that came out with more rules, and I had refused to sign it. At that point, I was willing to still stay and step, but I was not signing that manual. Two weeks after the conversation with the manager, I was removed from the step group chat.

I said to myself, *Ok. I'm not with them anymore. I'm going to need to do my own thing.*

It's time to rebrand.

Chapter 11
THE REBRAND

The rebrand was a challenge, but I felt empowered. I finally had the freedom to do everything I couldn't do before. That included being able to stamp my name on my board, whereas before, the previous company I stepped for only allowed their brand logo on the stepboards. Additionally, I chose my brand colors, created my logo, got my EIN, LLC, and registered my trademark. *I'm really doing this!* I thought. I was so excited to be independent. I didn't have a team to guide me. I didn't have anyone to teach me anything about building my own brand. I went to CapCut and Canva and figured out my marketing. A friend pointed out how all over the place my Instagram page was, and I noticed how put-together my old trainer's was. I decided to take a page from his book and make sure I showed up on my platform. If I wanted visibility, posting twice a week wasn't going to cut it. Whenever my feet hit the board, I had someone film me so I could get content and build my YouTube page. I knew how important it was for people to see me outside of the old brand I had been stepping with. I had already removed all of my old information with their logo, so it was time to replace everything with mine. I included my brand color purple in every single post.

My posts became purposeful and intentional. I was diving into brand storytelling. But even before all of that, I had to let my old trainer know about my new move. I never wanted to come between him and his brother, but he was totally understanding and supported me 100%. "I left them and I'm doing my own thing," I informed him. "Well done," he responded, and that rush of pleasure I always felt when he applauded me was back. He was so supportive he would even post me stepping on his social media platform.

Doing the rebrand was the first time in my life that I dove into the deep waters of entrepreneurship, and it was time to see if I would sink or swim. Regardless of the outcome, I believed in myself enough to try.

There were definitely some lonely times. The rebrand showed me who was for me and who wasn't. There were many I thought would be there to support me that I found out were instead gossiping behind my back. When I launched my own thing, sadly, a lot of folks were watching and waiting for me to fail. Haters said, "She'll be done in a year." Even though it hurt, I could see why they thought so. Most who left to be independent didn't make it. But I've been doing this for almost three years now. I made it.

Whenever someone says I can't do something, pride rises in me. *How dare you?!* I say back. *How dare you tell me I can't be a successful Black woman? How dare you say I need to abort my child? How dare you say I can't have my own step brand? I can and I will. Period.*

Even with my tenacity, every entrepreneur knows the grueling battle of standing alone. I would go to teach class, and it would be just one person, and that one person and I would step. Often, I dreaded going into my Tuesday class. There were too many times I would have to swallow my pride and embarrassment because a class would be packed before my class. Then once my class started, only two people would stay. I had to learn by staying and teaching those two people. I learned commitment. I learned discipline. I learned patience.

Success is never overnight. No one ever became a millionaire or super successful by showing up just one time. No. They show up through the good, the bad, *and* the ugly.

I even learned resilience in dealing with my abuser. Once he started doing step, we would be in the same classes, and sometimes, I would be stepping right next to him! When I would try to move away, he would only follow me. I could have whined and cried about it, but instead, I took it on the chin and kept stepping. Step taught me so much about myself, what I could handle, and that many others would be influenced by my purpose.

During the hard parts of building my brand, I would cry out to God for my tribe. Slowly, they started coming. One good friend, Drina, would step with me, and sometimes, it was just me and her. Then Debreona, AKA "23", Ms. Tracy, and Asia. I started building a foundation of steppers that would represent what the Ari brand stood for. These women would motivate me when it was hard to motivate myself. For so long I struggled with not feeling like a "girl's girl," because I related to guys more easily. But finally, I had women who had my back, and I found my clique. I became a "girl's girl" through the rebrand.

Outside of my initial steppers, there were others God would use. There were days I was depressed and wanted to give up. *I shouldn't go today,* I would think. *This is my last class,* I would promise myself when I didn't see the numbers, or when people said my class was too hard, too fast, and too advanced. But every time, God would use someone to keep me going. "Ari, you're the reason I got certified," someone DM'd me one day when I was struggling. "Keep going!" That happened four different times. I would be ready to throw in the towel and someone would pop up.

Chapter 11

There would be three of us on the floor, I would walk off and take a deep breath, and someone would walk behind me. "I love how you step, Ari. You're a great instructor. Keep going."

Ok. One more month, God, I would think, and then, it kept being one more month.

One particular message really encouraged me. The woman who sent it quoted Galatians 6: 7-9 "Whatever a man sows he shall reap." She said, "You *have* to reap!" and it hit me so hard. I had never heard of reaping being referred to as a positive thing. It was often used as a threat for something negative to happen. Her sharing that shifted my mindset, and I thought, *Yea! If I'm doing the right thing with this, I have to reap the good!* What made it even more meaningful is that the woman ended up becoming one of my core steppers. She joined me within a year of my rebrand.

Early in the process of building, I mustered up the courage to go live on YouTube on Wednesdays. I figured if the brand I stepped for could take off with five people in a basement, mine could too. I didn't need a full class to be noticed. And guess what? I was right. I started getting re-shares on social media. People started supporting outside of the fitness community I had previously left. That was so needed because it had become clear that my leaving the old brand had hindered my partnerships with many of their instructors. There would be times when instructors would reach out to step with me and then have to renege because the manual said they couldn't. I realized quickly I would need to find new step communities to link with.

Ok, so this rebrand will have to be a real *rebrand.*

Instead of deterring me, that hindrance only motivated me. I would go on social media pages of steppers and comment or remix their step and tag them or mirror their routine and tag them. They would say, "You're that Step Girl!" I started traveling to support them. My steppers and I would go out of town just to support someone, and a month later, I would be partnering with them to teach a class. That's how I started building a new step community. It was a lot of grit and grind, but I loved it.

The hard work started paying off. About a year after stepping under my brand, I went viral on a video where I stepped alone doing an advanced move. My platform grew by 5,000 followers off that one video! *Ok, God, this is confirmation.* That's when I really started being more in tune with what I was posting. I branched out of just posting about fitness and started posting about me. Before that post went viral all these people had never even heard of me. Now I could tell them who I was. I shared about all the things I was passionate about like autism, domestic violence, mental health, nutrition, spiritual health, eating disorders, and body dysmorphia. Social media became my diary, and, unintentionally, I began building community through my authenticity and transparency. I go viral on my son all the time from what I share online!

Though my popularity was increasing while instructing and growing my brand, my weight would fluctuate. I wasn't as thin as that 148lb. woman stepping in the basement five days a week. I was 163lbs. which was still small, but I was very aware of the weight gain. Bulimia is just like any other addiction and surfaced during this time of me gaining. It's still tempting even now, though I'm not acting on the temptation. *Should I throw up?* I often think after a meal. *It's just for this one time,* is always in the back of my mind. It's so hard.

One time, I looked up a support group, but they were extreme. *I don't need to be admitted for a month, I just need someone to talk to,* I thought. *These girls are still in their season of bulimia.* I had overcome my season, but I needed someone to talk about how hard it was not to go back. The struggle is real. I fell off a couple of times since I quit years ago, but both times I made myself sick, I felt horrible afterward. Thankfully, I wasn't in that space to get caught in that cycle again, but I don't know if the temptation will ever go away.

One thing that has helped with the battle of bulimia is being able to share my story and connect with others online who understand. One day, I went live on Instagram and talked about my bulimia. A nurse I graduated with, who had been a soccer player, commented on my live that she could relate. We ended up going live together and created a safe space for women in fitness to dialogue about these sensitive topics. It was so freeing and healing. I found the outlet I needed through creating it, just like I did with building my own step brand. To help with the weight gain, I got a personal trainer and took boxing classes which gave me a way to manage my ADHD, encourage my spirit, and help with my cardio burn.

While staying consistent and focusing on my brand and personal health, another pivotal moment came in my career. One of my good friends, Dee, is a fitness instructor and had been walking with me through the ups and downs of building my brand. She was such an inspiration on how she attracted her tribe, and I aimed to do the same. Dee came to me and said, "Ari, I'm going to be a part of 'Ebony Fit Weekend' and I'd like to put you on too." That was a huge opportunity! "Ebony Fit Weekend" is a wall-to-wall fitness conference that travels. That year in 2023, it was being held in Atlanta. Thanks to Dee, I was able to teach there, network, and partner with influencers and well-known fitness instructors after the event. That experience was a great confidence builder. I had been disappointed with seeing others steal my routines and not give me the credit, but this was motivation that there was a whole world of stepping outside of Cleveland, Ohio.

After the event, my email started blowing up with invitations. I was still travel nursing, so I limited myself to only doing out-of-town events once a month, but life was good. My classes started filling back up by me staying true to myself and my style. I kept stepping advanced and I attracted my people. I even started dating a really good guy. He DM'd me right after my rebrand, and we've been together ever since. This man is the healthiest man I've ever been with. He's supportive, patient, kind, and has nothing to do with the step or fitness world. It was so nice to meet someone who didn't already think they knew me based on my platform. Even when we started dating, he had no idea how popular I was. We would be out, and someone would approach me, "Hey! You're The Step Girl!" and he would be looking like, "What is going on?" He saw my social media pages and just thought I was a good stepper. It may seem strange, but his response made me happy. I didn't want someone who was with me for what I had done or how others perceived me to be. I wanted someone with me for me.

Regarding my professional growth, I continue searching for ways to expand. I started pressing my own clothes and selling fitness merchandise at events. I became contracted with Cuyahoga County to teach physical fitness to government employees. I started co-hosting an annual event called "Black March Madness" with Dee which is similar to "Ebony Fit Weekend" and gathers other fitness instructors to teach classes locally. In 2024, I even completed my instruction manual which allows me to certify step instructors. That was a major accomplishment. The way this came about was similar to how I became an instructor. People kept asking, "Ari, when are you going to certify other trainers?" I never felt worthy to, but realized that people were already learning from me indirectly and directly, so, why not? *If God did it for them, He can do it for me.*

My step instructor's manual includes rules that can benefit everyone. I wanted it to reflect excellence and foster communities that helped attendees thrive. It teaches how to hold a class, plus my originally created step moves, and requires CPR certification.

Now my focal point isn't to be the best stepper, it's to be the best instructor. I'm not worried about always having eyes on me; instead, I want to pass the torch. I want to create instructors who are of the same caliber as me; a group of high-functioning fitness people who feel good about themselves. They're awkward and not ashamed of doing too much. This is the place for them.

My brand's manual will be the answer to what I felt has been lacking in the step community. I believe we should step and be uniform but, at the same time, feel free to excel in our own style. This manual will help implement that belief. I never want anyone to feel how I felt in the back of that basement when the manager stopped liking me. I couldn't breathe. It was awful. I felt like I was being punished for being me. Now, I'm in a position to set the tone for my workout classes and certify others to model the environment I aim to reflect: a bully-free workout zone.

This way of doing things has helped the right people gravitate to me. I think people aren't just attracted to me because I do what I do so well but because I check on my people. I aim to be super down-to-earth, approachable for people to share their issues and a proactive leader. I connect with my steppers as individuals. I want everyone who comes to my class to know that they're valued and safe. It's not about perfection but about persistence. Success is about being consistent and disciplined. I attract those types of people. I attract people who are unapologetically themselves.

I look around now and smile. Many of the steppers who've come to me had been dealing with toxic workout spaces and came to my space for reprieve. They're all new faces and I love that for me. No one can say I'm a success because of the old brand I was with. I built this from the ground up. I also love that I see so much of myself in my core tribe of steppers. They're bubbly and happy and don't want drama. They're not competing. They just want to flow. But even when there are issues, I nip it in the bud fast. I know firsthand that one bad apple can ruin the whole bunch.

I've also had the pleasure of teaching steppers from scratch and seeing their growth. I've had so much fun creating step classes like "Bring Your Best Friend To Step Day" where the BFF gets in free. I gained a really great stepper from that class who I was able to groom from the beginning. Another core stepper who found out about me from out of town followed me on YouTube and now joins my classes regularly. In less than three years, the evolution and growth of my brand has blown my mind and I know there's more success on the way.

In my personal life, I'm happy. I'm working on me. Now my working out is more well-rounded. I lift weights. I box. I step. I do dance fitness. I do a variety of workouts. I'm not married to one thing. Though step is my passion, it's not my end-all-be-all anymore. I had to work on changing my mindset because I never wanted to be in that same position I was in with track, where, when something falls through, I don't have anything to fall back on. I never want to have to combat a loss of identity again because I can't do that one thing.

I'm still in this battle with food and constantly thinking about the contents of my food. *How many calories am I eating?* is always in the back of my mind. *Can I afford these calories?* Usually, it's an internal debate if I want to indulge. I can't remember the last time I wasn't concerned about my calorie count and I hope to one day not be in a position where I don't have to think about food all the time. It's exhausting. But even though I'm still in the fight, I'm grateful I'm not sick anymore. I spent years hating myself. I would be at the mall, catch a glimpse of my reflection in the mirror, and immediately look the other way. Or, I would see the long rows of mirrors attached to a store at the mall and go out of my way to avoid it. I used to loathe myself and my size. Now, I have more realistic expectations for my weight.

I battle every day not to let my anxiety and body dysmorphia keep me from purpose. I choose to show up authentic in every aspect of my journey and I think that's what brings the right energy into my life. I've learned from my mistakes. I've learned from choosing unhealthy relationships. My son is thriving. He's been with the same school for autistic children since he was seven years old. I couldn't be more proud of the teenager he is today.

At this point in my career, I realize that I've been perfectly and divinely aligned. All the people on my team came from me stepping out and taking a chance on myself. I bet on me and I won.

Looking back, I can see the rebrand was not just about step, it was about me. I had to say, "Ari, you're worth it. You can do this." Going through that negative experience of rejection in my workout community taught me to value my foundation. Treat your foundation with respect. Treat your "Day Ones" with respect and you can't help but win. *Period!*

Acknowledgments

Thank you, "Hoodie" (Robin). In 2022, you were the first person who told me I needed to write this book. You gave me the name and said to put a pun on the word "weight". I tried to write and couldn't get past the first paragraph, then met Nicole within months of you giving me that idea. God will align you! Thank you to my man Clarence Clayton. You are so supportive. Anytime I have rants, you listen. Anytime I have a vision, you say, "We will get it done." Thank you to my son for being my miracle baby and for keeping me aligned. Out of all the times I fell off, I always realigned myself because of you. Thank you to the father of my child. Thank you to my Day Ones (you know who you are) for rocking with me before it was cool to. I want to thank my old trainer for opening up your gym to me. A lot of my big events happened because you name-dropped me. I want to thank the head trainer I stepped for previously for sending me that text message that day. It changed my life. I was also so inspired by your hustle. I appreciate the opportunity to shine on your platform and even the shift for me to start my own. I want to thank the manager of the brand I used to step for. If you had never said to be an instructor, I would never be an instructor. Lastly, thank you to my mom for not just instilling discipline and organization in me, but for telling me I was worthy and beautiful early on, even when I wasn't ready to believe it.

www.ingramcontent.com/pod-product-compliance
Lightning Source LLC
Chambersburg PA
CBHW072213070526
44585CB00015B/1316